COLOR ATLAS & SYNOPSIS OF
CLINICAL OPHTHALMOLOGY
Ⅲ Wills Eye Institute

Pediatric
Ophthalmology

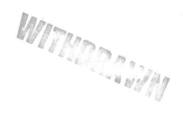

EDITOR
Leonard B. Nelson, MD, MBA
Co-Director, Pediatric Ophthalmology and Ocular Genetics
Wills Eye Institute
Associate Professor of Ophthalmology and Pediatrics
Jefferson Medical College of Thomas Jefferson University
Philadelphia, Pennsylvania

SECTION EDITORS
Michael J. Bartiss, OD, MD
Kammi B. Gunton, MD
Judith B. Lavrich, MD
Alex V. Levin, MD, MHSc
Scott E. Olitsky, MD
Jonathan H. Salvin, MD
Bruce M. Schnall, MD
Barry N. Wasserman, MD

SERIES EDITOR
Christopher J. Rapuano, MD
Director and Attending Surgeon, Cornea Service
Co-Director, Refractive Surgery Department
Wills Eye Institute
Professor of Ophthalmology
Jefferson Medical College of Thomas Jefferson University
Philadelphia, PA

COLOR ATLAS & SYNOPSIS OF CLINICAL OPHTHALMOLOGY

))) Wills Eye Institute

Pediatric Ophthalmology

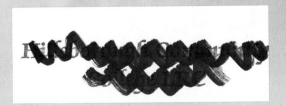

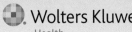 Wolters Kluwer | Lippincott Williams & Wilkins
Health

Philadelphia • Baltimore • New York • London
Buenos Aires • Hong Kong • Sydney • Tokyo

Senior Executive Editor: Jonathan W. Pine, Jr.
Senior Product Managers: Emilie Moyer and Grace Caputo
Senior Manufacturing Coordinator: Benjamin Rivera
Marketing Manager: Lisa Lawrence
Creative Director: Doug Smock
Production Services: Aptara, Inc.

© 2012 by LIPPINCOTT WILLIAMS & WILKINS, a Wolters Kluwer business
First edition, © 2003 The McGraw-Hill Companies, Inc.
Two Commerce Square
2001 Market Street
Philadelphia, PA 19103 USA
LWW.com

Printed in China

978-1-4511-1087-6
1-4511-1087-1
Library of Congress Cataloging-in-Publication Data
available upon request

Care has been taken to confirm the accuracy of the information presented and to describe generally accepted practices. However, the authors, editors, and publisher are not responsible for errors or omissions or for any consequences from application of the information in this book and make no warranty, expressed or implied, with respect to the currency, completeness, or accuracy of the contents of the publication. Application of the information in a particular situation remains the professional responsibility of the practitioner.

The authors, editors, and publisher have exerted every effort to ensure that drug selection and dosage set forth in this text are in accordance with current recommendations and practice at the time of publication. However, in view of ongoing research, changes in government regulations, and the constant flow of information relating to drug therapy and drug reactions, the reader is urged to check the package insert for each drug for any change in indications and dosage and for added warnings and precautions. This is particularly important when the recommended agent is a new or infrequently employed drug.

Some drugs and medical devices presented in the publication have Food and Drug Administration (FDA) clearance for limited use in restricted research settings. It is the responsibility of the health care provider to ascertain the FDA status of each drug or device planned for use in their clinical practice.

To purchase additional copies of this book, call our customer service department at (800) 638-3030 or fax orders to (301) 223-2320. International customers should call (301) 223-2300.

Visit Lippincott Williams & Wilkins on the Internet: at LWW.com. Lippincott Williams & Wilkins customer service representatives are available from 8:30 am to 6 pm, EST.

10 9 8 7 6 5 4 3 2 1

To my wife Helene for her understanding, patience, and support.
To my children, Jen, Kim, and Brad, who have taught me what is important in life.
To my son-in-law, Josh, who embodies the meaning of family.
To my two grandsons, Jake and Ryan, who never cease to amaze me.

And to the memory of several individuals who passed away recently and
who had a profound effect on my personal and professional life:
Dean Henry S. Coleman, whose extraordinary guidance through
my college years at Columbia University fine-tuned my future goals.
A. Stone Freedberg, MD, who was instrumental in my matriculating and
succeeding as a medical student at Harvard Medical School.
Marshall M. Parks, MD, who taught me pediatric ophthalmology and
whose skills in all aspects of the subspecialty I have always tried to emulate.

Editors

SERIES EDITOR

Christopher J. Rapuano, MD
Director and Attending Surgeon, Cornea Service
Co-Director, Refractive Surgery Department
Wills Eye Institute
Professor of Ophthalmology
Jefferson Medical College of Thomas Jefferson
    University
Philadelphia, PA

EDITOR

Leonard B. Nelson, MD, MBA
Co-Director, Pediatric Ophthalmology and Ocular
    Genetics
Wills Eye Institute
Associate Professor of Ophthalmology and
    Pediatrics
Jefferson Medical College of Thomas Jefferson
    University
Philadelphia, Pennsylvania

SECTION EDITORS

Michael J. Bartiss, OD, MD
Pinehurst, North Carolina

Kammi B. Gunton, MD
Department of Pediatric Ophthalmology and
    Ocular Genetics
Wills Eye Institute
Philadelphia, Pennsylvania

Judith B. Lavrich, MD
Department of Pediatric Ophthalmology and
    Ocular Genetics
Wills Eye Institute
Thomas Jefferson University Medical Center
Philadelphia, Pennsylvania

Alex V. Levin, MD, MHSc
Chief, Pediatric Ophthalmology and Ocular Genetics
Wills Eye Institute
Professor, Departments of Ophthalmology and
    Pediatrics
Jefferson Medical College of Thomas Jefferson
    University
Philadelphia, Pennsylvania

Scott E. Olitsky, MD
Professor of Ophthalmology
Chief, Section of Ophthalmology
Children's Mercy Hospitals and Clinics
University of Missouri—Kansas City School of
    Medicine
Kansas City, Missouri

Jonathan H. Salvin, MD
Division of Ophthalmology
Nemours/A.I. duPont Hospital for Children
Wilmington, Delaware
Clinical Assistant Professor
Departments of Pediatrics and Ophthalmology
Wills Eye Institute
Jefferson Medical College of Thomas Jefferson
    University
Philadelphia, Pennsylvania

Bruce M. Schnall, MD
Associate Surgeon
Department of Pediatric Ophthalmology and
    Ocular Genetics
Wills Eye Institute
Philadelphia, Pennsylvania
Clinical Associate Professor
Department of Surgery
UMDNJ—Robert Wood Johnson Medical School
Camden, New Jersey

Barry N. Wasserman, MD
Department of Pediatric Ophthalmology,
    Strabismus and Ocular Genetics
Wills Eye Institute
Philadelphia, Pennsylvania

Contributors

Alok S. Bansal, MD
Fellow, Vitreoretinal Surgery
Retina Service
Wills Eye Institute
Philadelphia, Pennsylvania

Hillary Gordon, BS
Jefferson Medical College
Philadelphia, Pennsylvania

Anuradha Ganesh, MD
Fellow, Pediatric Ophthalmology and Ocular
    Genetics
Wills Eye Institute
Philadelphia, Pennsylvania

Harold P. Koller, MD, FAAP, FACS
Professor of Ophthalmology
Thomas Jefferson University
Adjunct Professor of Ophthalmology
Drexel University College of Medicine
Attending Surgeon
Wills Eye Institute
Philadelphia, Pennsylvania

Carol L. Shields, MD
Professor of Ophthalmology
Thomas Jefferson University Hospital
Co-Director, Oncology Service
Wills Eye Institute
Philadelphia, Pennsylvania

Jerry A. Shields, MD
Professor of Ophthalmology
Thomas Jefferson University Hospital
Director of Oncology Service
Wills Eye Institute
Philadelphia, Pennsylvania

Anya A. Trumler
Fellow in Pediatric Ophthalmology and
    Ocular Genetics
Wills Eye Institute
Philadelphia, Pennsylvania

About the Series

The beauty of the atlas/synopsis concept is the powerful combination of illustrative photographs and a summary approach to the text. Ophthalmology is a very visual discipline that lends itself nicely to clinical photographs. Although the seven ophthalmic subspecialties in this series—Cornea, Retina, Glaucoma, Oculoplastics, Neuroophthalmology, Pediatrics, and Uveitis—use varying levels of visual recognition, a relatively standard format for the text is used for all volumes.

The goal of the series is to provide an up-to-date clinical overview of the major areas of ophthalmology for students, residents, and practitioners in all of the health care professions. The abundance of large, excellent quality photographs and concise, outline-form text will help achieve that objective.

Christopher J. Rapuano, MD
Series Editor

Preface

Wills Eye Institute has been my "academic home" for over 30 years. During that time, I have witnessed remarkable changes in pediatric ophthalmology as it has become a more established and rapidly expanding subspecialty. Although many changes have occurred at Wills over those years, certain things have remained constant, including the outstanding faculty, fellows, residents, and staff, as well as the commitment to excellent patient care and academic endeavors. Wills is a rich storehouse of clinical material and has provided the major background for this book. In particular, the Pediatric Ophthalmology and Ocular Genetics Department at Wills, which cares for thousands of children each year, provides a rare opportunity for the study of an extremely wide variety of pediatric ocular disorders. It has been a pleasure to oversee the production of this book as each contributor has been part of the "Wills family."

The advances that have occurred in the understanding of pediatric ocular disease and newer modalities of treatment require a constant updating of knowledge about these conditions. This text was written in an effort to provide practicing ophthalmologists, pediatric ophthalmologists, and residents in training with a concise update of the clinical findings and the most recent treatment available for a wide spectrum of childhood ocular diseases. The disorders are grouped according to the specific ocular structure involved. The atlas format should provide readers with a clear and succinct outline of the disease entities and stimulate a more detailed pursuit of the specific ocular disorders.

Leonard B. Nelson, MD, MBA
Editor

Acknowledgments

It is with pleasure and gratitude that I acknowledge a number of individuals who helped make this publication possible. I appreciate the members of the Audio-Visual Department at Wills Eye Institute, Roger Barone and Jack Scully, who helped in the preparation of many of the photographs. I am grateful to Peg Savino for her exceptional secretarial skills. I am indebted to Grace Caputo, the developmental editor, for her continuous suggestions and help throughout the preparation of this book. Finally, I wish to thank all the authors who gave of their time, unselfishly, in the writing of this book.

The editors would also like to acknowledge the fine work of Dr. Rizwan Alvi in the preparation of this book.

Contents

Editors   vi

Contributors   vii

About the Series   viii

Preface   ix

Acknowledgments   x

CHAPTER 1 **Abnormalities Affecting the Eye as a Whole   2**

Judith B. Lavrich

Anophthalmia   2
Microphthalmia   8
Nanophthalmia   12
Typical Coloboma   14

CHAPTER 2 **Congenital Corneal Opacity   18**

Bruce Schnall and Michael J. Bartiss

Sclerocornea   18
Birth Trauma: Tears in Descemet's Membrane   20
Ulcer or Infection   22
Mucopolysaccharidosis   24
Peters' Anomaly   26
Congenital Hereditary Endothelial Dystrophy   28
Corneal Dermoid   30
Anterior Staphyloma   32
Wilson's Disease (Hepatolenticular Degeneration)   34
Herpes Simplex Infection   36
    Herpes Simplex Virus Epithelial Dendrite or Ulceration   38
    Herpes Simplex Virus Corneal Stromal Disease   40
Herpes Zoster Ophthalmicus   42
Chickenpox   44
Limbal Vernal Keratoconjunctivitis   46

CHAPTER 3 **Glaucoma   48**

Alex V. Levin and Anya A. Trumler

Primary Congenital or Infantile Glaucoma   48
Juvenile Open-Angle Glaucoma   52
Aphakic Glaucoma   55
Uveitic Glaucoma   58
Sturge-Weber Syndrome   62

Congenital Ectropion Uveae 65

Aniridia 68

Posterior Embryotoxon 70

CHAPTER 4 **Iris Anomalies 72**

Michael J. Bartiss and Bruce M. Schall

Central Pupillary Cysts (Pupillary Margin Epithelial Cysts) 72

Aniridia 74

Brushfield Spots 76

Ectopia Lentis et Pupillae 78

Heterochromia Iridis 80

Iris Coloboma 82

Iris Stromal Cysts 84

Juvenile Xanthogranuloma 86

Lisch Nodules 88

Melanosis Oculi (Ocular Melanocytosis) 90

Persistent Pupillary Membrane 92

Posterior Synechiae 94

Axenfeld-Rieger Anomaly 96

CHAPTER 5 **Lens Anomalies 98**

Jonathan H. Salvin and Hillary Gordon

Congenital and Developmental Cataracts 98

Ectopia Lentis 102

Anterior Lenticonus 104

Posterior Lenticonus 106

Spherophakia 108

CHAPTER 6 **Retinal Anomalies 110**

Barry N. Wasserman, Anuradha Ganesh, Alex V. Levin,
Carol L. Shields, Jerry A. Shields, and Alok S. Bansal

Best's Disease 110

Choroideremia 112

Gyrate Atrophy 114

Leber Congenital Amaurosis 116

Astrocytic Hamartoma 118

Incontinentia Pigmenti 120

Coats' Disease 124

Retinoblastoma 128

Congenital Hypertrophy of the Retinal Pigment Epithelium 134

Familial Exudative Vitreoretinopathy 136

Persistent Fetal Vasculature 138

Juvenile Retinoschisis 140

Retinopathy of Prematurity 142

Retinitis Pigmentosa   146
Myelinated Nerve Fibers   148
Stargardt's Disease or Fundus Flavimaculata   150

CHAPTER 7 **Eyelid Anomalies   152**

Kammi B. Gunton

Ankyloblepharon   152
Blepharophimosis Syndrome   154
Congenital Ectropion   156
Congenital Entropion   158
Congenital Ptosis   160
Eyelid Colobomas   162
Epiblepharon   164
Epicanthus   166
Capillary Hemangiomas   168

CHAPTER 8 **Lacrimal Anomalies   170**

Leonard B. Nelson and Harold P. Koller

Congenital Mucocele   170
Congenital Nasolacrimal Duct Obstruction   172

CHAPTER 9 **Strabismus Disorders   174**

Scott E. Olitsky and Leonard B. Nelson

Pseudoesotropia   174
Congenital (Infantile) Esotropia   176
Inferior Oblique Overaction   178
Dissociated Vertical Deviation   179
Refractive Accommodative Esotropia   180
Nonrefractive Accommodative Esotropia   181
Nonaccommodative or Partially Accommodative Esotropia   182
Congenital Exotropia   183
Intermittent Exotropia   184
A and V Pattern Strabismus   185
Third Nerve Palsy   188
Fourth Nerve Palsy   190
Sixth Nerve Palsy   192
Duane's Syndrome   194
Brown's Syndrome   196
Möbius Syndrome   198
Monocular Elevation Deficiency   200
Congenital Fibrosis of the Extraocular Muscles   202

Index   205

COLOR ATLAS & SYNOPSIS OF CLINICAL OPHTHALMOLOGY

Wills Eye Institute

Pediatric Ophthalmology

Abnormalities Affecting the Eye as a Whole

Judith B. Lavrich ■

ANOPHTHALMIA

Anophthalmia, also known as anophthalmos, is a congenital anomaly that is characterized by the complete absence of ocular tissue within the orbit. **Primary** or **true anophthalmia** is a very rare condition and can involve one or both eyes. Extreme microphthalmos is far more common and can be mistaken for this condition. Anophthalmia has a prevalence of 0.18 per 10,000 births and has no racial or sexual predilection.

Etiology

During embryogenesis, there is an arrest in the development of the neuroectoderm of the primary optic vesicle, which stems from the anterior neural plate of the neural tube.

Anophthalmia is most frequently idiopathic and sporadic but can be inherited as a dominant, recessive, or sex-linked trait. It is associated with maternal infections during pregnancy (e.g., toxoplasmosis, rubella) as well as syndromes with craniofacial malformations (e.g., Goldenhar, Hallerman-Streiff, Waardenburg syndromes). It is linked with genetic defects, including trisomies 13 to 15; chromosomal deletion in band 14q22-23 with associated polydactyly; and deletions involving SOX2, SIX6, and STRA6.

Signs

- The eye is the stimulus for proper growth of the orbital region; therefore, an infant born with anophthalmia has the following:
  - Orbital findings
    - ▶ Small orbital rim and entrance
    - ▶ Reduced size of bony orbital cavity
    - ▶ Globe is completely absent
    - ▶ Extraocular muscles are usually absent
    - ▶ Lacrimal gland and ducts may be absent
    - ▶ Small or maldeveloped optic foramen
  - Eyelid findings
    - ▶ Narrow palpebral fissures
    - ▶ Foreshortening of the eyelids
    - ▶ Shrunken conjunctival fornices
    - ▶ Levator function is decreased or absent with poor eyelid folds
    - ▶ Contracture of the orbicularis oculi muscle

Symptoms

- Unilateral or bilateral blindness because of absence of the globe(s)

Differential Diagnosis

- Microphthalmos, which includes:

  - Secondary anophthalmos: the development of the eye begins but gets arrested, resulting in only residual eye tissue or extreme microphthalmos.

  - Degenerative anophthalmos: there is formation of the optic vesicle, but subsequent degeneration occurs from lack of blood supply or other causes.

- Cryptophthalmos: abnormal fusion of the entire eyelid margin with absence of the eyelashes

- Cystic eye: a cyst of neuroglial tissue lacking normal ocular structures

Diagnostic Evaluation

- Anomalous eyelid and orbital features (Fig. 1-1)

- Ultrasound imaging. B-scan ultrasonography of the orbit will show a complete absence of the globe. After 22 weeks' gestation, transvaginal ultrasonography can detect eye malformations but its sensitivity in the detection of anophthalmia is not known.

- Magnetic resonance imaging (MRI) scan of the head and orbits. MRI will show the soft tissue within the orbital cavity (Fig. 1-2). Associated intracranial abnormalities can also be evaluated. Individuals with bilateral anophthalmos may have a related hypoplastic or absent optic chiasm as well as agenesis or dysgenesis of the corpus callosum.

- Computed tomography (CT) scan of the head and orbits. CT scan will image the bony changes and intracranial and craniofacial abnormalities seen with anophthalmia.

Treatment

- Medical care

  - Orbital conformers can be placed in the orbital cavity to stimulate growth of the bony orbit (Fig. 1-3). As the orbit grows, the conformers are changed and progressively increased in size to further expand the orbital cavity. This serial augmentation takes time and cooperation from both the patient and parents.

  - Contraction and reversal of the benefit often occur if the conformer is left out of the orbit for a significant amount of time. With unilateral anophthalmos, the family should be aware that, most likely, the final result will not mirror the normal healthy orbit.

  - An ocular prosthesis can be fitted over the conformer to simulate the eye and improve appearance.

- Surgical care

  - The small bony cavity is both a cosmetic deformity and may not allow proper fitting of a prosthesis. Therefore, surgery may be indicated for either of these problems.

  - Inflatable tissue expanders are used if conformers are not well tolerated or cannot be fit. The inflatable silicone expander is surgically positioned deep in the orbit and is accessed through a tube placed at the lateral orbital rim. The expander is filled with saline and gradually reinflated on a weekly or biweekly schedule. Compared with solid conformers, inflatable expanders may allow more rapid and extensive expansion of the bony orbit. When the desired volume is achieved, the port and bladder need to be removed and replaced with a permanent implant.

  - Hydrogel (methylmethacrylate and N-vinylpyrrolidone) expanders are self-expanding hydrophilic expanders that are implanted in the orbital tissue in their dry, contracted state through a small incision. The implant gradually expands in size by osmotic absorption of surrounding tissue fluid. The benefit of this method is the controlled self-expansion, reducing the risk of tissue atrophy, and without the need for repeat fittings or surgery.

■ Dermis fat grafting involves biocompatible grafts that grow slowly over time can be a good option to restore volume to the hypoplastic orbit. The graft is harvested from a second surgical site, typically the buttocks. However, the graft compatibility and growth can be variable. In some cases, the fat can atrophy. Rarely, the fat can hypertrophy, necessitating debulking.

■ Injectable calcium hydroxylapatite (Radiesse) is a semipermanent dermal filler that has been reported as a new, simple, cost-effective technique to treat volume deficiency in the anophthalmic orbit in adults. Augmentation is accomplished with serial injections of the filler until adequate volumization is achieved. The results have demonstrated a lasting effect in the orbit of 1 year or more.

■ Orbito-cranial advancement surgery is used for orbital expansion if conformers and expanders are unsuccessful. This method involves multiple osteotomies to divide the periocular bones and advancing them forward and outward with bone grafts and plates.

■ Because the foreshortening of the eyelids may limit the passage of a large conformer, a lateral canthotomy or cantholysis may be needed to increase the horizontal length of the palpebral fissure. Other methods to lengthen the eyelids may include skin, mucosal, or cartilage grafts.

Prognosis

● Severe cosmetic deformities can result from anophthalmia, especially if not treated early. Even with proper treatment, the results are often cosmetically suboptimal with incomplete expansion of the orbit, malformations and immobility of the eyelids, and complete immobility of the ocular prosthesis.

● Psychosocial issues caused by absence of an eye and facial disfigurement can result. Referral for psychological counseling may be indicated for these children.

REFERENCES

Bardakiian T, Weiss A, Schneider AS. Anophthalmia/microphthalmia overview. In Pagon RA, Bird TC, Dolan CR, Stephens K, eds. *GeneReviews.* Seattle: University of Washington; 2007:1993–2004.

Bernardino R. Congenital anophthalmia: A review of dealing with volume. *Middle East Afr J Ophthalmol.* 2010;17:156–160.

http://www.geneclinics.org/profiles/anophthalmia-ov/index.html.

Verma AS, Fitzpatrick DR. Anophthalmia and microphthalmia. *Orphanet J Rare Dis.* 2007;2:47.

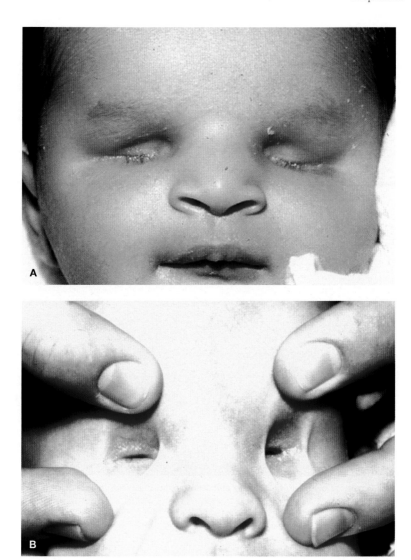

FIGURE 1-1. **A.** External examination of bilateral anophthalmia. **B.** Clinical examination of bilateral anophthalmia showing empty orbits. (Courtesy of Leonard B. Nelson, MD.)

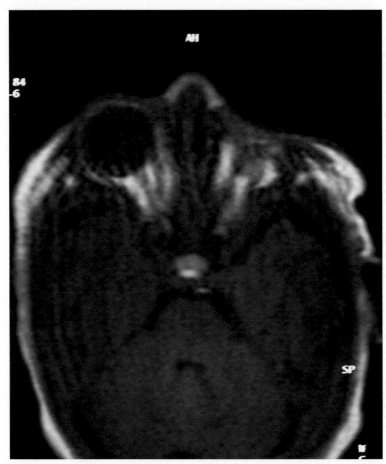

FIGURE 1-2. Magnetic resonance image showing unilateral anophthalmia with absence of the globe. (Courtesy of Carol Shields, MD.)

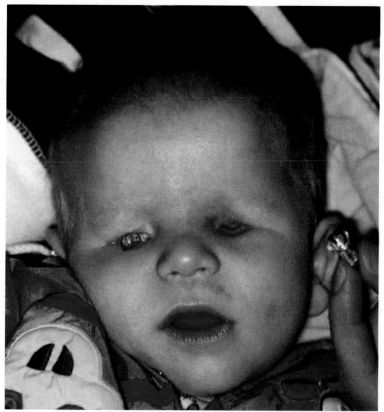

FIGURE 1-3. Fitting orbital conformers in bilateral "clinical anophthalmia" (severe microphthalmia). (Courtesy of Bruce Schnall, MD.)

MICROPHTHALMIA

Microphthalmia is a congenital unilateral or bilateral condition in which the globe has a reduced axial length that is at least two standard deviations below the mean for age. The appearance of the globe and the severity of axial length reduction define the classification of microphthalmia:

● **Simple or pure microphthalmia:** an eye that is anatomically intact except for its short axial length. Simple microphthalmia is suspected in the presence of high hyperopia (≥8 diopters) or microcornea. Visual loss can occur in a subset of microphthalmos associated with posterior segment abnormalities.

● **Severe microphthalmia:** an eye that is severely reduced in size, with an axial length less than 10 mm at birth or less than 12 mm after age one and a corneal diameter less than 4 mm (**Fig. 1-4**). The globe may be inconspicuous on clinical examination, but remnants of ocular tissue, an optic nerve, and extraocular muscles will be seen with imaging.

● **Complex microphthalmia:** a globe with reduced size associated with developmental ocular malformations of the anterior or posterior segment (or both).

There are two types of microphthalmos: noncolobomatous and colobomatous (microphthalmos with cyst) (**Fig. 1-5**). The prevalence of microphthalmia is 1.5 per 10,000 births. There is no racial or sexual predilection.

Etiology

● Microphthalmia results from an arrest in the development at any stage during the growth of the optic vesicle.

  ■ Environmental: prenatal exposure of alcohol, thalidomide, retinoic acid, or rubella

  ■ Heritable: via autosomal dominant, recessive, or X-linked inheritance

  ▶ Multiple chromosomal abnormalities

  ▶ Single-gene disorders causing syndromic microphthalmia (e.g., CHARGE [coloboma of the eye or central nervous system anomalies, heart defects, atresia of the choanae, retardation of growth or development, genital or urinary defects, and ear anomalies or deafness], Lenz microphthalmia, Goltz, Aicardi, Walker-Warburg and Meckel-Gruber syndrome, Norrie disease, incontinentia pigment)

  ▶ Other genes: *SIX3, HESX1, SHH, CHX10, RAX*

  ■ Unknown causes: Goldenhar syndrome; cases associated with basal encephalocele and other central nervous system anomalies

Signs

● Significant variability exists depending on the severity of the microphthalmos.

  ■ Orbital findings

    ▶ Small orbital rim and entrance

    ▶ Reduced size of bony orbital cavity

    ▶ Globe is extremely small and can be malformed

    ▶ Extraocular muscles are present but are usually hypoplastic

    ▶ Lacrimal gland and ducts are present but are usually hypoplastic

    ▶ Optic nerve is present but is usually hypoplastic

    ▶ Small or maldeveloped optic foramen

  ■ Eyelid findings

    ▶ Narrow palpebral fissures

    ▶ Foreshortening of the eyelids

    ▶ Shrunken conjunctival fornices

    ▶ Levator function is decreased or absent with poor eyelid folds

    ▶ Contracture of the orbicularis oculi muscle

Symptoms

- The extent of visual loss depends of the severity of the microphthalmos and the presence of related anomalies.

Differential Diagnosis

- Microcornea with a normal-sized globe
- High hyperopia

Diagnostic Evaluation

- Anomalous eyelid and orbital features
- Clinical examination looking for evidence of a cornea or globe
  - Palpation of the orbit to estimate globe size
  - Measurement of corneal diameter (normal range, 9.0–10.5 mm in neonates)
- B-scan ultrasonography to evaluate the internal structures of the globe (Fig. 1-6A)
- CT scan or MRI of the brain and orbits to evaluate the size of the globe and its internal structures, the presence of optic nerve and extraocular muscles, and brain anatomy (Fig. 1-6B and C)

Treatment

- For severe microphthalmia, the treatment is the same as for anophthalmia.
- For simple or complex microphthalmos with vision
  - Treatment of amblyopia: patching of the healthy eye to stimulate as much potential vision as possible
  - Protection of the healthy eye in children with unilateral involvement
  - Visual aids and other visual resources for children with reduced vision
  - Orbital conformers: placed over the microphthalmic eye to stimulate growth of the bony orbit. These can be painted or with the pupil left clear for vision.
  - Ocular prosthesis: can be fitted over the globe to improve appearance, if needed

Prognosis

- For severe microphthalmia, the prognosis is the same as for anophthalmia.
- For simple microphthalmia, the visual prognosis depends on the severity of the condition and the associated ocular abnormalities.

REFERENCES

Bardakiian T, Weiss A, Schneider AS. Anophthalmia/microphthalmia overview. In Pagon RA, Bird TC, Dolan CR, Stephens K, eds. *GeneReviews*. Seattle: University of Washington; 2007:1993–2004.

Bernardino R. Congenital anophthalmia: A review of dealing with volume. *Middle East Afr J Ophthalmol.* 2010;17:156–160.

http://www.geneclinics.org/profiles/anophthalmia-ov/index.html.

Verma AS, Fitzpatrick DR. Anophthalmia and microphthalmia. *Orphanet J Rare Dis.* 2007;2:47.

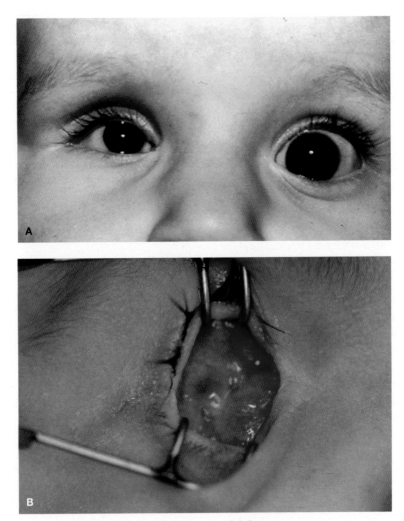

FIGURE 1-4. **A.** Unilateral microphthalmia. **B.** Severe microphthalmia.

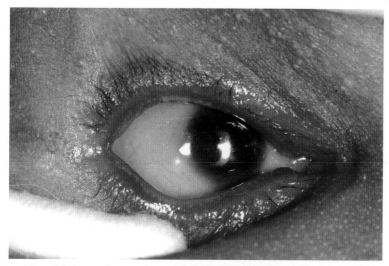

FIGURE 1-5. Microphthalmia with a cyst. (Courtesy of Carol Shields, MD.)

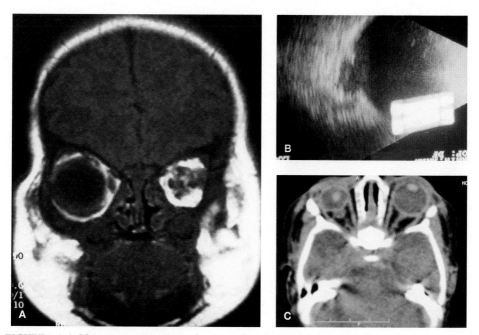

FIGURE 1-6. **A.** Magnetic resonance image showing unilateral microphthalmia. Note the presence of extraocular muscles and an optic nerve. **B.** B-scan ultrasonography scan of microphthalmia with a cyst showing a posterior staphyloma. **C.** Computed tomography scan of microphthalmia with a cyst showing disorganization of ocular tissues and posterior cyst. (Courtesy of Carol Shields, MD.)

NANOPHTHALMIA

Nanophthalmia is a subtype of simple microphthalmia. It is a congenital and typically bilateral condition (Fig. 1-7), although can be unilateral. It is characterized by reduced globe volume, although the eye is otherwise grossly normal.

Etiology

• Nanophthalmia results from an arrest in the growth of the eye during the embryonic stage and may result from a smaller optic vesicle anlage.

• Most cases are sporadic, but both autosomal recessive and autosomal dominant inheritance have been reported.

Signs

• Reduced axial length of the globe (<20 mm)

• Very high hyperopia (>10 diopters)

• Reduced corneal diameter

• Lens is normal in size

• Shallow anterior chamber

• Thick sclera

• Fundus may show crowded optic disc, vascular tortuosity, and macular hypoplasia

• Because of the anatomy, these eyes have a high risk for angle-closure glaucoma. They tolerate intraocular surgery poorly with a high rate of complications, including uveal effusion and retinal detachment.

Differential Diagnosis

• High hyperopia in a normal eye

Diagnostic Evaluation

• Measurement of corneal diameter

• A-scan to measure the axial length of the eye

• Pentacam and ultrasound biomicroscopy to image the anterior chamber and assess its depth (Fig. 1-8).

Treatment

• Management of narrow-angle or angle-closure glaucoma is initially medical, although the response to treatment is typically poor, and miotics may even worsen the condition by relaxing the lens zonules. Peripheral laser iridotomy may be moderately successful. Caution must be used with fistulizing glaucoma surgery because postoperative malignant glaucoma can ensue. Laser trabeculoplasty, if performed, must be done early before permanent damage to the outflow mechanism occurs.

• Removal of the lens must be anticipated and can be complicated by uveal effusion and nonrhegmatogenous retinal detachments. Although challenging in these high-risk eyes, small-incision cataract surgery is safe and diminishes the need for prophylactic sclerotomies.

Prognosis

• The prognosis for vision is good if glaucoma is treated early and successfully.

REFERENCES

Bardakiian T, Weiss A, Schneider AS. Anophthalmia/microphthalmia overview. In Pagon RA, Bird TC, Dolan CR, Stephens K, eds. *GeneReviews*. Seattle: University of Washington; 2007:1993–2004.

Bernardino R. Congenital anophthalmia: A review of dealing with volume. *Middle East Afr J Ophthalmol.* 2010;17:156–160.

http://www.geneclinics.org/profiles/anophthalmia-ov/index.html.

Sharan S, Grigg JR, Higgins RA. Nanophthalmos: Ultrasound biomicroscopy and Pentacam assessment of angle structures before and after cataract surgery. *J Cataract Refract Surg.* 2006;32:1052–1055.

Verma AS, Fitzpatrick DR. Anophthalmia and microphthalmia. *Orphanet J Rare Dis.* 2007;2:47.

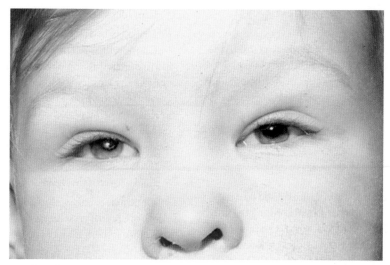

FIGURE 1-7. Bilateral nanophthalmia. Note the reduced corneal diameter.

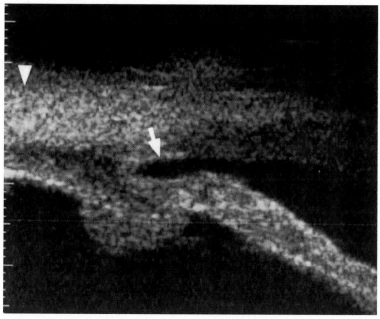

FIGURE 1-8. Ultrasound biomicroscopy of the anterior chamber in nanophthalmos. The iris is bowed forward, creating a plateau-like configuration of the narrow angle (*arrow*), and the anterior sclera (*arrowhead*) shows increased thickness. (From Buys YM, Pavlin CJ. Retinitis pigmentosa, nanophthalmos, and optic disc drusen: a case report. *Ophthalmology.* 1999;106:619–622.)

TYPICAL COLOBOMA

The term *coloboma* is derived from the Greek *koloboma*, meaning mutilated or curtailed. It is a congenital malformation and refers to a notch, gap, hole, or fissure in any of the ocular structures. Typical colobomas are frequently bilateral and are often associated with microphthalmia.

Etiology

- "Typical" colobomata are caused by defective closure of the optic fissure during the fifth to seventh weeks of fetal life and because of the location of the fetal fissure, are found in the inferonasal quadrant in the eye. ("Atypical" colobomata are less frequent malformations located outside the inferotemporal quadrant, for which the etiology is still unclear.)

- Most cases are idiopathic and sporadic, but all types of inheritance (i.e., autosomal dominant, autosomal recessive, and X-linked) have been reported and may be associated with various syndromes, such as CHARGE, Meckel-Gruber, Lenz microphthalmia, Aicardi, Patau, and Edwards syndromes. The prevalence of coloboma is 0.7 per 10,000 births.

Signs

- Ocular colobomata may affect any of the structures or the entire globe traversed by the fetal fissure from the iris to the optic nerve. It has a variable appearance depending on the extent and severity of the coloboma.

  - Iris: transillumination defect, heterochromia iridis, "teardrop" pupil (**Fig. 1-9A**)

  - Lens: defect or flattening of lens or absence of lens zonules inferiorly

  - Chorioretina: thinning of the choriocapillaris; pigment clumping along the line of optic fissure closure; colobomatous defect usually with sharp edges and circumscribed by irregular pigmentation; white sclera is seen through defect if all layers of chorioretina are absent; floor of defect sometimes bulges forming staphyloma

  - Leukocoria: if the uveal defect is large

  - Optic nerve: enlarged, excavated, vertically oval; retinal vessels may radiate in a spoke-like fashion from the nerve (**Fig. 1-9B and C**)

  - Globe: microphthalmia in some cases

  - Vision: ranges from normal to no light perception

- May be associated with a variety of other developmental defects.

Differential Diagnosis

- Atypical coloboma
- Retinal toxoplasmosis
- Optic nerve pits
- Morning glory syndrome
- Optic nerve hypoplasia

Diagnostic Evaluation

- Clinical examination of the eye

Treatment

- Patching for amblyopia: if unilateral with optic nerve involvement to stimulate as much potential vision as possible

- Treat ocular complications: cataract, subretinal neovascularization, retinal breaks or detachment

Prognosis

- Vision depends on involvement of the optic nerve, macula, and papulomacular bundle. However, visual acuity cannot be predicted from either coloboma size or optic nerve involvement because patients with large colobomata with optic nerve involvement can have almost normal vision.

REFERENCES

Chang L, Blain D, Bertuzzi S, et al. Uveal coloboma: clinical and basic science update. *Curr Opin Ophthalmol.* 2006;17:447–470.

Onwochei BC, Simon JW, Bateman JB, et al. Ocular colobomata. *Surv Ophthalmol.* 2000;45:175–194.

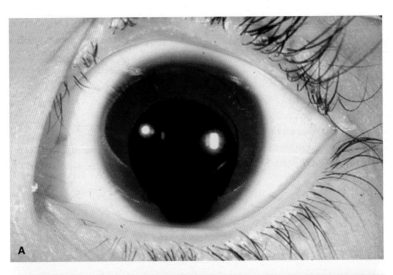

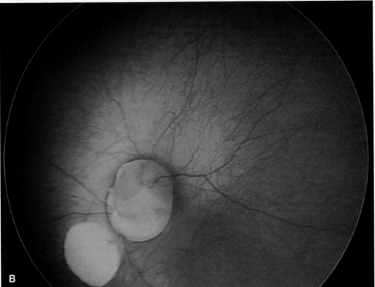

FIGURE 1-9. A. Iris coloboma. **B.** Coloboma involving the retina and optic nerve showing an enlarged optic nerve and radiating retinal vessels.

(*continued*)

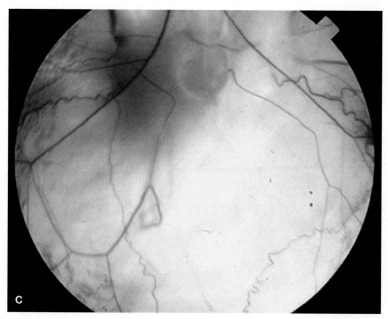

FIGURE 1-9. (*Continued*) **C.** Extensive chorioretinal and optic nerve coloboma. Note the round, yellow-appearing optic nerve and the significant disorganization of the tissues.

Congenital Corneal Opacity

Bruce Schnall and Michael J. Bartiss ■

The differential diagnosis for congenital corneal opacity can be remembered using the pneumonic STUMPED:

Sclerocornea

Tears in Descemet's membrane or birth trauma

Ulcer or infection

Mucopolysaccharidosis (MPS)

Peters' anomaly

Endothelial dystrophy, congenital hereditary (CHED)

Dermoid

SCLEROCORNEA

Etiology

● Developmental anomaly of the cornea

● Defective mesodermal migration during embryogenesis, resulting in tissue resembling sclera rather than clear corneal stroma

● Can be autosomal dominant, recessive, or sporadic

● Has been associated with the 22q11.2 deletion syndrome

Symptoms

● Opacified cornea present since birth

Signs

● Usually bilateral but can be unilateral

● Opacification of the cornea with the peripheral cornea more opacified than the central cornea (Fig. 2-1)

● May have fine blood vessels

Differential Diagnosis

● Tears in Descemet's membrane or birth trauma

● Ulcer or infection

● MPS

● Peters' anomaly

● CHED

● Dermoid

● Glaucoma

Treatment

● Evaluation by a genetic specialist to look for associated congenital anomalies

● If the central cornea is clear, it can be associated with cornea plano and a high refractive error.

- Penetrating keratoplasty should be considered if the central visual axis is involved and the posterior segment is relatively normal.

Prognosis

- Visual outcome with or without keratoplasty depends on the presence of other ocular and systemic abnormalities.

REFERENCES

Binenbaum G, McDonald-McGinn DM, Zackai EH, et al. Sclerocornea associated with the chromosome 22q11.2 deletion syndrome. *Am J Med Genet A.* 2008; 146(7):904–909.

Doane JF, Sajjadi H, Richardson WP. Bilateral penetrating keratoplasty for sclerocornea in an infant with monosomy 21. Case report and review of the literature. *Cornea.* 1994;13(5):454–458.

Kim T, Cohen EJ, Schnall BM, et al. Ultrasound biomicroscopy and histopathology of sclerocornea. *Cornea.* 1998;17(4):443–445.

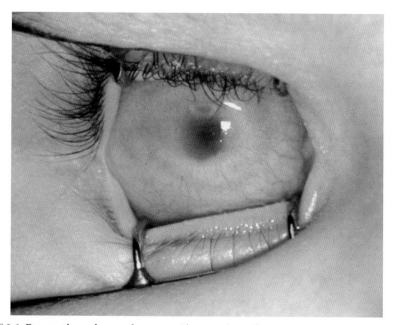

FIGURE 2-1. Descemet's membrane: sclerocornea. The corneal opacification is more severe peripherally than centrally.

BIRTH TRAUMA: TEARS IN DESCEMET'S MEMBRANE

Etiology

- Trauma to the cornea during vaginal delivery resulting in tears in Descemet's membrane
- May be associated with the use of forceps

Symptoms

- Corneal edema or opacification present at birth, which may resolve within the first few days of life

Signs

- Unilateral corneal edema or opacification present at birth (Fig. 2-2A)
- Often observed to have eyelid swelling and evidence of trauma to eyelids at birth
- Corneal edema often resolves within the first few days of life, revealing the Descemet's membrane ruptures, which usually appear as vertical linear tears (Fig. 2-2B and C). Descemet's tears associated with congenital glaucoma are usually oriented horizontally or curvilinearly (Fig. 2-3).
- Multiple tears are often present.
- Associated with high astigmatism

Differential Diagnosis

- Sclerocornea
- Ulcer or infection
- MPS
- Peters' anomaly
- CHED
- Dermoid
- Glaucoma

Treatment

- Descemet's tears are associated with high astigmatism, which is amblyogenic. Treatment of the amblyopia includes correction of the refractive error with glasses or contacts and part-time occlusion of the fellow eye.
- Penetrating keratoplasty should be considered if the corneal edema does not resolve.

Prognosis

- Visual outcome depends on the success of amblyopia treatment.

REFERENCE

Lambert SR, Drack AV, Hutchinson AK. Longitudinal changes in the refractive errors of children with tears in Descemet's membrane following forceps injuries. *J AAPOS.* 2004;8(4):368–370.

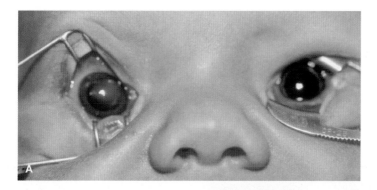

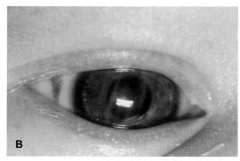

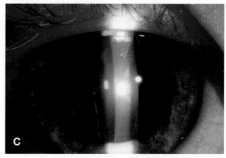

FIGURE 2-2. **A.** Corneal opacification in a newborn from Descemet's tears associated with birth trauma. **B.** The vertically oriented linear Descemet's membrane ruptures can now be seen in the same infant a few days later after the corneal edema has cleared. **C.** The vertically oriented Descemet's membrane breaks from birth trauma can be seen in this older child at the slit lamp with retroillumination.

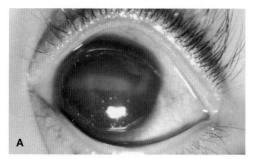

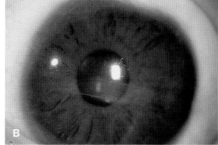

FIGURE 2-3. **A.** Recent Descemet's membrane ruptures associated with glaucoma. Note that the breaks are oriented horizontally. They are recent and therefore have overlying corneal edema. **B.** Breaks in Descemet's membranes caused by glaucoma. The horizontally oriented breaks can be seen more clearly after resolution of the corneal edema.

ULCER OR INFECTION

Etiology

- Acquired bacterial or herpetic infection

Symptoms

- Acquired corneal opacity usually associated with conjunctival injection and eyelid swelling (Fig. 2-4)

Signs

- Usually unilateral
- Corneal opacity with overlying epithelial defect
- Associated with conjunctival injection and other signs of inflammation
- May have associated systemic infection
- May have associated eyelid lesions or eyelid abnormalities

Differential Diagnosis

- Sclerocornea
- Tears in Descemet's membrane or birth trauma
- MPS
- Peters' anomaly
- CHED
- Dermoid
- Glaucoma

Treatment

- Depends on underlying cause or organism
- Prompt systemic treatment may be needed

Prognosis

- May result in a visually significant corneal scar

REFERENCE

Luchs JI, Laibson PR, Stefanyszyn MA, et al. Infantile ulcerative keratitis secondary to congenital entropion. *Cornea.* 1997;16:1:32–34.

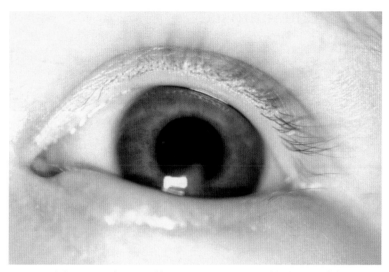

FIGURE 2-4. Corneal ulcer in an infant caused by congenital entropion of the lower eyelid.

MUCOPOLYSACCHARIDOSIS

Etiology

- Inborn error of metabolism
- Enzyme deficiency leads to a block in a metabolic pathway, which results in accumulation of material in the cornea.

Symptoms

- Acquired opacification of the cornea:
  - Hurler's syndrome, or MPS 1H, is associated with corneal clouding by 6 months of age
  - Scheie's syndrome, or MPS 1S, is associated with corneal clouding by 12 to 24 months of age

Signs

- Acquired corneal cloudiness or haze (Fig. 2-5)
- Associated systemic features (coarse facial features, mental retardation, poor growth, deafness)

Differential Diagnosis

- Sclerocornea
- Tears in Descemet's membrane or birth trauma
- Ulcer or infection
- Peters' anomaly
- CHED
- Dermoid
- Glaucoma

Diagnosis

- Evaluation by a genetic specialist
- Urine testing for MPS
- Enzyme assay
- Gene testing for gene defect

Treatment

- Enzyme replacement
- Bone marrow transplant

Prognosis

- Depends on severity of systemic disease and success of systemic treatment

REFERENCE

Kenyon KR, Navon SE, Haritoglou C. In: Krachmer JH, Mannis MJ, Hollane EJ, eds. *Cornea*. 2nd ed. Vol 1. Philadelphia: Elsevier Mosby; 2005: 749–776.

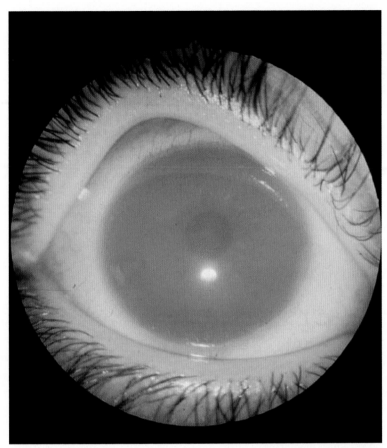

FIGURE 2-5. Hurler's syndrome. Note the generalized corneal haze. (Courtesy of Alex Levin, MD.)

PETERS' ANOMALY

Etiology

- Congenital
- Can be autosomal dominant, recessive, or sporadic
- May be associated with mutation of the *PAX6* gene

Symptoms

- Central corneal opacity present at birth (Fig. 2-6)
- 80% are bilateral.

Signs

- Central corneal leukoma with adherent iris strands (Fig. 2-7)
- Adherent iris strands usually originate from the iris collarette to the posterior surface of the corneal leukoma.
- May have associated cataract and glaucoma

Differential Diagnosis

- Sclerocornea
- Tears in Descemet's membrane or birth trauma
- Ulcer or infection
- MPS
- CHED
- Dermoid
- Glaucoma

Diagnosis

- Examination under anesthesia may be needed to confirm diagnosis and rule out glaucoma.

Treatment

- Evaluation by a genetic specialist to look for associated anomalies and to rule out Peters' plus syndrome
- Treat glaucoma if present.
- Penetrating keratoplasty should be considered within the first few months of life if the central visual axis is involved and posterior segment is relatively normal.
- If a visually significant cataract is present, cataract removal may be needed.

Prognosis

- Depends on involvement of the anterior segment; prognosis is poorer if a cataract or glaucoma is present
- Depends on success of amblyopia treatment
- Early keratoplasty may reduce amblyopia.

REFERENCES

Mailette De Buy Wenniger-Prick LJ, Hennekam RC. The Peters' plus syndrome: a review. *Ann Genet.* 2002;45(2):97–103.

Yang LL, Lambert SR, Drews-Botsch C, et al. Long-term visual outcome of penetrating keratoplasty in infants and children with Peters anomaly. *J AAPOS.* 2009;13(2):175–180.

Yang LL, Lambert SR, Lynn MJ, et al. Long-term results of corneal graft survival in infants and children with Peters anomaly. *Ophthalmology.* 1999; 106(4):833–848.

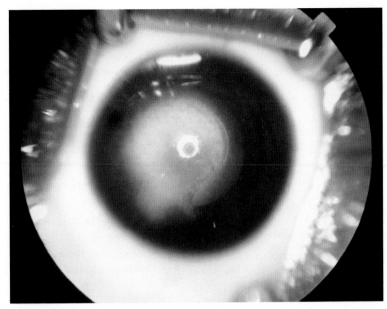

FIGURE 2-6. Peters' anomaly. Note the central opacity and the clear corneal periphery.

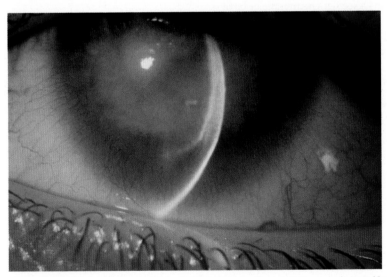

FIGURE 2-7. Slit-lamp photograph of Peters' anomaly. Note the iris adherent to the central corneal leukoma. (Courtesy of Alex Levin, MD.)

CONGENITAL HEREDITARY ENDOTHELIAL DYSTROPHY

Etiology

- Congenital
- Can be autosomal dominant, recessive, or sporadic

Symptoms

- Corneal haze present since birth (Fig. 2-8)

Signs

- Bilateral symmetrical corneal edema
- Swollen, thickened cornea with minimal epithelial edema
- Rarely associated with glaucoma

Differential Diagnosis

- Sclerocornea
- Tears in Descemet's membrane or birth trauma
- Ulcer or infection
- MPS
- Peters' anomaly
- Dermoid
- Glaucoma

Diagnosis

- CHED can be confused with congenital glaucoma
- Corneal thickness two to three times normal
- Examination under anesthesia may be needed to confirm corneal thickening and to rule out glaucoma.

Treatment

- Mild edema can be treated with hypertonic saline solutions.
- Penetrating keratoplasty is usually needed if corneal haze is significant. Descemet stripping endothelial keratoplasty may be an alternative to penetrating keratoplasty.

Prognosis

- Depends on graft survival and amblyopia
- Early keratoplasty may reduce amblyopia.

REFERENCES

Javadi MA, Baradaran-Rafii AR, Zamani M, et al. Penetrating keratoplasty in young children with congenital hereditary endothelial dystrophy. *Cornea.* 2003; 22(5):420–423.

Mittal V, Mittal R, Sangwan VS. Successful Descemet stripping endothelial keratoplasty in congenital hereditary endothelial dystrophy. *Cornea.* 201;30(3): 354–656.

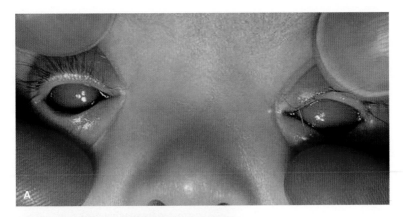

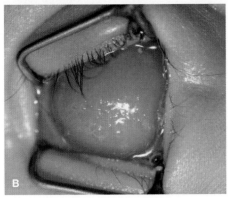

FIGURE 2-8. Congenital hereditary endothelial dystrophy (Courtesy of Alex Levin, MD.)

CORNEAL DERMOID

Etiology

- Developmental anomaly of the cornea
- Limbal dermoids may be associated with Goldenhar's syndrome, also known as faciao auricular vertebral syndrome and oculo-auriculo-vertebral dysplasia.

Symptoms

- Corneal opacity present since birth

Signs

- Domelike mass of the cornea
- Most commonly located at the corneal limbus (epibulbar dermoid) but can be located centrally (Fig. 2-9)
- May contain hairs or fatty tissue (lipodermoids)
- Normal intraocular pressure (IOP) and corneal diameter

Differential Diagnosis

- Sclerocornea
- Tears in Descemet's membrane or birth trauma
- Ulcer or infection
- MPS
- Peters' anomaly
- CHED
- Glaucoma

Treatment

- Often associated with astigmatism, which will result in amblyopia
- Patching and correction of refractive error may be needed to treat amblyopia.
- Some corneal or limbal dermoids can be treated by shaving flush with corneal surface or lamellar keratoplasty.
- Penetrating keratoplasty can be considered if the central visual axis is involved.

Prognosis

- Visual outcome depends on success of amblyopia treatment.

REFERENCES

Arora R, Jain V, Mehta D. Deep lamellar keratoplasty in corneal dermoid. *Eye (Lond)*. 2005;19(8):920–921.

Mansour AM, Barber JC, Reinecke RD, et al. Ocular choristomas. *Surv Ophthalmol*. 1989;33(5):339–358.

Watts P, Michaeli-Cohen A, Abdolell M, et al. Outcome of lamellar keratoplasty for limbal dermoids in children. *J AAPOS*. 2002;6(4):209–215.

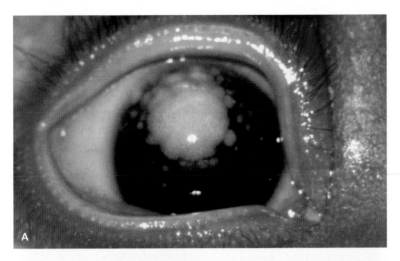

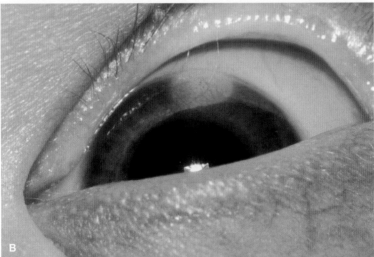

FIGURE 2-9. **A.** Centrally located corneal dermoid. Note the satellite-like lesions. **B.** Dermoid located at the limbus superiorly.

ANTERIOR STAPHYLOMA

Etiology

- Developmental anomaly of the anterior segment

Symptoms

- Bulging opacified cornea

Signs

- Bulging or protuberant congenital corneal opacity that may prevent the eyelids from closing fully
- Can be unilateral or bilateral (Fig. 2-10)
- Cornea usually thinned and enlarged

Differential Diagnosis

- Sclerocornea
- Tears in Descemet's membrane or birth trauma
- Ulcer or infection
- MPS
- Peters' anomaly
- CHED
- Dermoid

Treatment

- Often treated with evisceration or enucleation (Fig. 2-11)
- Corneoscleral transplant can be considered.

Prognosis

- Visual prognosis is poor.

REFERENCES

Lunardelli P, Matayoshi S. Congenital anterior staphyloma. *J Pediatr Ophthalmol Strabismus.* 2009;25: 1–2.

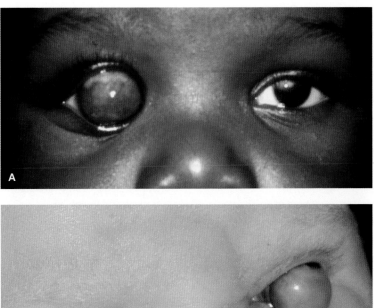

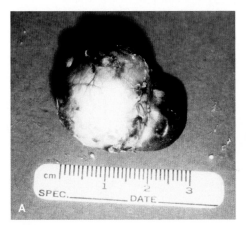

FIGURE 2-10. A. Unilateral anterior staphyloma. **B.** Bilateral anterior staphyloma.

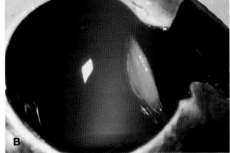

FIGURE 2-11. Enucleation specimen of anterior staphyloma. **A.** Gross specimen of enucleated eye with anterior staphyloma, note the bulging cornea. **B.** Specimen showing view of lens and anterior staphyloma to the right of the lens.

WILSON'S DISEASE (HEPATOLENTICULAR DEGENERATION)

Etiology

- Autosomal recessive inherited disorder caused by multiple allelic substitutions or deletions in the DNA coding for B-polypeptide, Cu^{++} transporting and ATPase
- Defect linked to chromosome 13q14.3-q21.1
- Systemic decreased level of ceruloplasmin causing decreased ability to properly transport copper
- Copper deposition in liver and kidneys followed by brain and Descemet's membrane

Symptoms

- Muscular rigidity, tremor, and involuntary movements (can resemble Parkinson's disease)
- Speech difficulties and dementia also occur.

Signs

- Golden brown, red, or green ring of pigmentation (known as Kayser-Fleischer ring) at the level of the posterior lamella of Descemet's membrane (Fig. 2-12)
- Usually begin at the 12- and 6-o'clock positions in the cornea and spread circumferentially around the cornea
- May be several millimeters thick

Differential Diagnosis

- Intrahepatic cholestasis of childhood
- Biliary cirrhosis
- Chronic active hepatitis

Treatment

Kayser-Fleischer rings gradually disappear with successful treatment.

- D-penicillamine (works via chelating Cu^{++} ions)
- British anti-Lewisite (BAL)
- Copper-deficient diet
- Liver transplantation

Prognosis

- Studies have shown retinal electrophysiological abnormalities improving with successful treatment.

REFERENCES

Liu M, Cohen EJ, Brewer GJ, Laibson PR. Kayser-Fleischer ring as the presenting sign of Wilson disease. *Am J Ophthalmol.* 2002;133(6):832–834.

Slovis TL, Dubois RS, Rodgerson DO, Silverman A. The varied manifestations of Wilson's disease. *J Pediatr.* 1971;78(4):578–584.

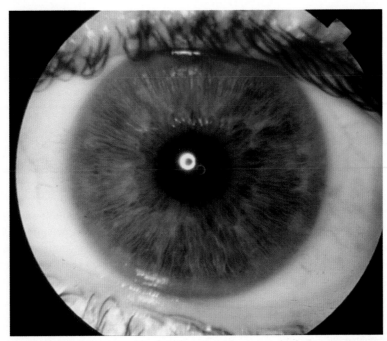

FIGURE 2-12. Kayser-Fleisher ring in a patient with Wilson's disease. Note the brown-red ring in the periphery of the cornea.

HERPES SIMPLEX INFECTION

Etiology

- Infection with herpes simplex virus (HSV) type 1 or 2
- Usually acquired during childhood, occasionally acquired during the birth process
- Ocular infection with HSV can affect the eyelids, conjunctiva, or cornea.
- HSV blepharoconjunctivitis

Symptoms

- Vesicular lesions on the eyelid or red inflamed eye
- Vesicles cross the dermatomes and progress to crusting (Fig. 2-13).
- Usually unilateral
- May be recurrent

Signs

- Clear vesicles with an erythematous base
- Often associated with an enlarged preauricular lymph node on the affected side

- Conjunctival involvement results in conjunctival injection and eyelid swelling.
- May be associated with a conjunctival dendrite, which is best seen at the slit lamp with fluorescein

Differential Diagnosis

- Herpes zoster ophthalmicus: Rash is dermatomal and does not cross the midline.

Diagnosis

- Based on characteristic clinical findings
- In atypical cases, diagnosis can be confirmed by viral cultures, polymerase chain reaction (PCR) testing, or the appearance of multinucleated giant cells on Giemsa staining of scrapings.

Treatment

- Topical (trifluridine drops or ganciclovir ophthalmic gel) or of systemic (acyclovir or valacyclovir) antiviral agents (or both topical and systemic agents may be used).
- Long-term oral antiviral prophylaxis is recommended for children with multiple recurrent episodes.

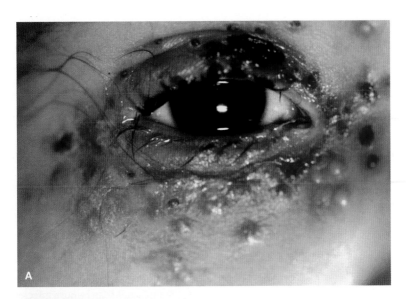

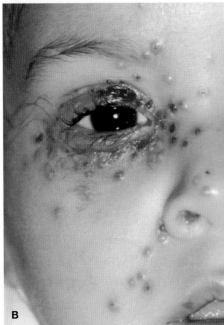

FIGURE 2-13. Herpes simplex blepharitis. **A.** Vesicular lesions, some of which are now crusted. **B.** The vesicular lesions cross dermatomes.

HERPES SIMPLEX VIRUS EPITHELIAL DENDRITE OR ULCERATION

Symptoms

- Red, painful eye
- Tearing, photophobia, decreased vision
- History of previous HSV infection
- Usually unilateral

Signs

- Dendrite that appears as a linear branching epithelial defect with terminal bulbs (Fig. 2-14A)

- May appear as a geographic ulceration (Fig. 2-14B)

- Epithelial edges of herpetic lesions are swollen and stain intensely

Diagnosis

- Based on characteristic clinical findings

- In atypical cases, diagnosis can be confirmed by viral cultures, PCR testing, or the appearance of multinucleated giant cells on Giemsa staining of corneal scrapings.

Treatment

- Topical (trifluridine drops or ganciclovir ophthalmic gel) or of systemic (acyclovir or valacyclovir) antiviral agents (or both topical and systemic agents may be used)

- Consider cycloplegics for significant photophobia or uveitis is present.

- Debridement can remove infected epithelium.

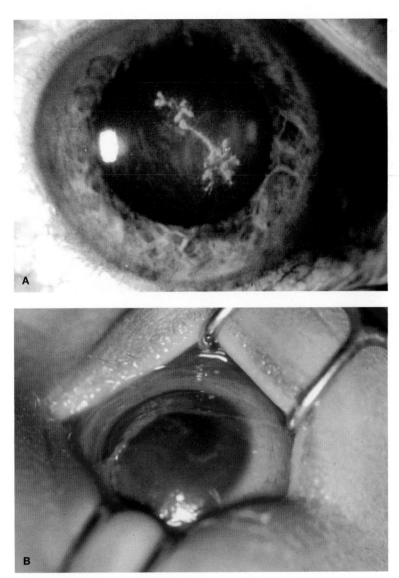

FIGURE 2-14. A. Herpes simplex corneal dendrite. The dendrite stains with fluorescein when viewed with cobalt blue light. (Courtesy of Alex Levin, MD.) **B.** Herpes simplex geographic corneal ulcer in an infant. Note the white, raised leading edge of the ulcer.

HERPES SIMPLEX VIRUS CORNEAL STROMAL DISEASE

Symptoms

- Unilateral corneal opacity (Fig. 2-15)
- Red, painful eye
- Tearing, photophobia, decreased vision
- History of previous HSV infection

Signs

- Disciform keratitis (Fig. 2-16A)
  - Disc-shaped stromal opacity
  - Intact epithelium
  - Mild anterior chamber reaction
  - Keratopercipitates are common
- Interstitial keratitis (Fig. 2-16B)
  - Multiple or diffuse white stromal infiltrates
  - Neovascularization or ghost vessels

Diagnosis

- Based on characteristic clinical findings
- Decreased corneal sensation

Treatment

- Combination of antiviral agents and steroids

REFERENCES

Chong EM, Wilhelmus KR, Matoba AY, et al. Herpes simplex virus keratitis in children. *Am J Ophthalmol.* 2004; 138(3):474–475.

Hsiao CH, Yeung L, Yeh LK, Kao LY, et al. Pediatric herpes simplex virus keratitis. *Cornea.* 2009;28(3): 249–253.

Schwartz GS, Holland EJ. Oral acyclovir for the management of herpes simplex virus keratitis in children. *Ophthalmology.* 2000;107(2):278–282.

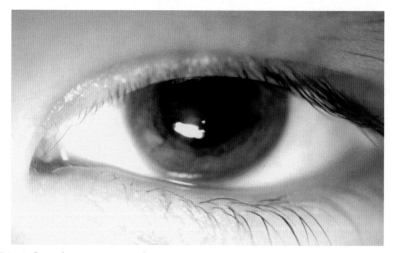

FIGURE 2-15. Corneal opacity in an uninflamed eye months after herpes simplex infection.

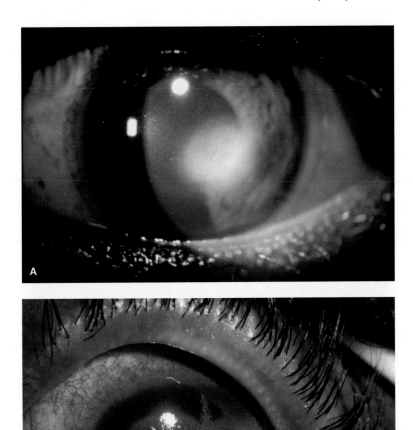

FIGURE 2-16. **A.** Active herpes simplex interstitial keratitis. **B.** Disciform keratitis. Note the disclike corneal haze seen in the slit-lamp photograph.

HERPES ZOSTER OPHTHALMICUS

Etiology

- Reactivation of latent varicella (chicken-pox virus) from cranial nerve ganglia

- More common in the elderly population but may occur if the child had chickenpox in utero or within the first 6 months of life

- Has occurred in children immunized for chickenpox

- Can occur in individuals who are immunocompromised

Symptoms

- Unilateral vesicular lesions associated with pain

- May be preceded by headache or neuralgia in affected dermatome

Signs

- Vesicular rash isolated to the dermatome of the fifth cranial nerve (Fig. 2-17)

- Rash usually respects the midline

- May develop conjunctivitis, small epithelial dendrites (pseudodendrites), disciform keratitis, and uveitis

- Corneal disease and uveitis skin may not begin till several days to weeks after the onset of the skin eruption

Differential Diagnosis

- Herpes simplex: Rash is not dermatomal and crosses the midline.

Diagnosis

- Based on characteristic clinical findings and associated skin vesicles

Treatment

- Systemic antivirals if within 4 days of onset of skin eruptions

- Analgesics may be needed to treat associated pain.

- Conjunctivitis and pseudodendrites can be treated with lubrication.

- Disciform keratitis and uveitis are treated with topical steroids.

REFERENCE

De Freitas D, Martins EN, Adan C, et al. Herpes zoster ophthalmicus in otherwise healthy children. *Am J Ophthalmol.* 2006;142(3):393–399.

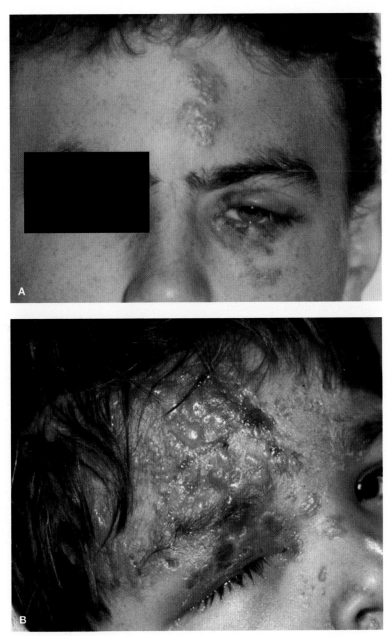

FIGURE 2-17. Herpes zoster ophthalmicus. Note the dermatomal distribution of the vesicles (**A** and **B**) and the significant eyelid edema (**B**).

CHICKENPOX

Etiology

- Primary infection with varicella (chickenpox virus)

Symptoms

- Disseminated vesicular lesions that affect the skin and mucous membranes

- Red eye, conjunctival lesion (Fig. 2-18)

Signs

- Conjunctival vesicle or ulceration

- Less commonly may develop superficial punctate keratitis, dendrite without terminal bulbs, or disciform keratitis

- Often associated with a transient mild anterior uveitis but can trigger a persistent uveitis that requires treatment

Diagnosis

- Based on characteristic clinical findings and associated skin vesicles

Treatment

- Self-limited conjunctivitis

- Topical antibiotics may prevent secondary bacterial infection.

Prognosis

- Usually resolves without conjunctival or corneal scarring

REFERENCE

Pavan-Langston D. In: Smolin G, Thoft RA, eds. *The Cornea*. Boston: Little, Brown and Company; 1983:189.

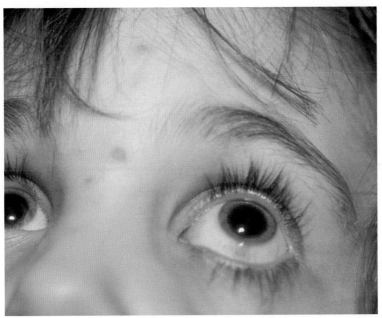

FIGURE 2-18. Chickenpox lesion can be seen just inferior to the cornea in the left eye and on the face.

LIMBAL VERNAL KERATOCONJUNCTIVITIS

Etiology

- Most common cause is seasonal allergies

Symptoms

- Elevated gelatinous mass along the corneal limbus
- Red, itchy eyes
- Mucous production

Signs

- Discrete gray-white nodules at cornea limbus. These nodules have a whitish center that is filled with eosinophils (Horner-Trantas dots; Fig. 2-19).
- The nodules may become confluent.
- Conjunctiva surrounding these nodules is injected.
- Usually bilateral, but involvement may be asymmetrical.

Diagnosis

- Based on characteristic clinical findings
- History of seasonal allergies

Treatment

- Topical antihistamine and mast cell stabilizers
- Topical steroids may be needed; best used in pulsed doses. When using topical steroids, careful monitoring, including monitoring IOP, is needed to prevent steroid side effects.
- Oral antihistamines and removal of suspected allergens can be helpful.

REFERENCE

Krachmer JH, Mannis MJ, Hollane EJ, eds. *Cornea*. 2nd ed. Vol 1. Philadelphia: Elsevier Mosby; 2005:552–558.

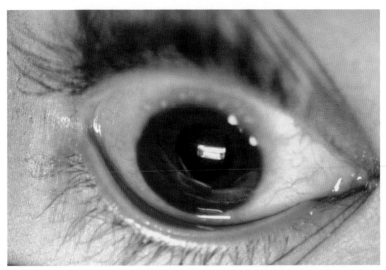

FIGURE 2-19. Limbal vernal. White, elevated lesions (Horner-Trantas dots) can be seen along the corneal limbus superiorly.

Glaucoma

Alex V. Levin and Anya A. Trumler ▪

PRIMARY CONGENITAL OR INFANTILE GLAUCOMA

Glaucoma diagnosed within the first four years of life and not associated with other findings of anterior segment dysgenesis. When present at birth, it is called *congenital glaucoma* Characteristic findings include buphthalmos, corneal enlargement, Haab striae (breaks in Descemet's membrane), increasing axial length, anterior iris insertion on gonioscopy, and corneal edema.

Epidemiology and Etiology

- The incidence of primary congenital or infantile glaucoma varies in different populations of the world with a reported incidence of 1 in 10,000 in the United States. It has a much higher incidence in Saudi Arabia and Gypsies of Romania (one in 2500 and one in 1250, respectively), with both populations having a higher rate of consanguinity.

- Most commonly, mutations in the *CYP1B1* (2p21) gene, which encodes a cytochrome P450 protein, are the cause. Two other genes and at least one other locus have been identified. In the Arabic and Gypsy population, a homozygous mutation in *CYP1B1* has been found in more than 94% of cases, suggesting an autosomal recessive inheritance. In isolated cases, the frequency of *CYP1B1* mutation decreases to 10% to 15%.

- The pathogenesis of primary congenital or infantile glaucoma remains elusive. The theory of an imperforate membrane (Barkan's membrane) over the trabecular meshwork is controversial. The patients clearly have a gonio-dysgenesis, which likely represents a failure of complete neural crest differentiation, resulting in impaired aqueous outflow. Clinically, the angle is characterized on gonioscopy as a high flat or patchy high insertion with absence of the angle recess and iris inserting directly on the trabecular meshwork (Fig. 3-1).

History

- Primary congenital or infantile glaucoma is bilateral in 75% of cases, which can create a delay in diagnosis because parents may simply believe their child has "beautiful big eyes."

- The classic symptom triad is photophobia, epiphora, and blepharospasm. Buphthalmic eyes with corneal stromal or epithelial edema (Fig. 3-2) is often the presenting sign.

- Elevated IOP causes stretching of the cornea with resultant breaks in Descemet's membrane, called Haab striae (Fig. 3-3). The stretching of the anterior segment also gives the sclera a blue appearance because of the underlying hue of the uvea.

Signs

- Characteristic findings include increased IOP, optic nerve cupping, corneal enlargement, Haab striae, increasing axial length, and gonioscopy findings (see Diagnostic Evaluation section).

Differential Diagnosis

- Congenital hereditary endothelial dystrophy (CHED)
- Congenital hereditary stromal dystrophy (CHSD)
- Mucopolysaccharidosis
- Sclerocornea or Peters' anomaly
- Keratitis
- Forceps birth trauma
- Megalocornea
- Contralateral microphthalmia
- Nasolacrimal duct obstruction

Diagnostic Evaluation

- A patient with corneal clouding, increased corneal diameter, and optic nerve cupping should raise the suspicion for primary congenital or infantile glaucoma and prompt further evaluation with an examination under anesthesia, including biomicroscopy, pachymetry, corneal diameter measurement, gonioscopy, refraction, axial length measurement, and (if possible) optic nerve photography.
- When measuring intraocular pressure (IOP) under anesthesia, attention should be paid regarding the type of anesthetic agent used. Whereas ketamine increases IOP measurements, halothane significantly lowers IOP, as do other anesthetic agents but to a lesser extent.

- Corneal hysteresis should be taken into account because corneal edema falsely lowers the IOP measurements. Asymmetry of IOP of 5 mm Hg is also an important indication of an abnormality.

- The normal corneal diameter in an infant younger than 1 year of age is 11 mm, with a corneal diameter greater than 12 mm, asymmetry between the eyes, and significant progression over time all being suggestive of primary congenital or infantile glaucoma.

- Retinoscopy and axial length measurement using immersion A-scan provides objective measurements to suggest increased axial length. The mean axial length at birth is 17 mm and increases to 20 mm by 1 year of age.

Treatment and Prognosis

- Medical management with antiglaucoma medications in primary congenital or infantile glaucoma is used as a temporizing agent, with definitive treatment being surgical.

- Antiglaucoma medications, including carbonic anhydrase inhibitors (both topical and oral), low-dose beta-blockers, and prostaglandins, may be used to clear the cornea for surgical intervention. Brimonidine should not be used in infants younger than the age of 1 year because there is a risk of potentially life-threatening apnea, hypotension, bradycardia, and hypothermia.

- The primary procedure of choice in primary congenital or infantile glaucoma is goniotomy or trabeculotomy depending on the preference of the surgeon and adequate visualization of anterior chamber angle that is needed for goniotomy. Both have reported short-term success rates of 60% to 90%. In one epidemiologic study, goniotomy offered a long-term cure in only 48.7% of patients. In patients who have failed goniotomy or trabeculotomy, secondary surgery may include goniosurgery on the remaining angle or trabeculectomy or glaucoma drainage device.

- The goal of primary congenital or infantile glaucoma treatment is more than achieving a normal IOP but more importantly attaining and maintaining normal visual function. Aggressive treatment of refractive error, amblyopia, and visually significant optical opacities are an important component to the infant's care. Lifelong follow-up of these patients is needed to monitor for glaucoma progression. Optic nerve cupping in infants is reversible and is a hallmark of successful glaucoma management. The most common cause of visual loss is amblyopia.

REFERENCES

Bejjani BA, Lewis RA, Tomey KF, et al. Mutations in CYP1B1, the gene for cytochrome P4501B1, are the predominant cause of primary congenital glaucoma in Saudi Arabia. *Am J Hum Genet.* 1998;62:325–333.

Curry SM, Daou AG, Hermanns P, et al. Cytochrome P4501B1 mutations cause only part of primary congenital glaucoma in Ecuador. *Ophthalmic Genet.* 2004;25:3–9.

Debnath SC, Teichmann KD, Salamah K. Trabeculectomy versus trabeculotomy in congenital glaucoma. *Br J Ophthalmol.* 1989;73:608–611.

Gencik A. Epidemiology and genetics of primary congenital glaucoma in Slovakia. Description of a form of primary congenital glaucoma in gypsies with autosomal-recessive inheritance and complete penetrance. *Dev Ophthalmol.* 1989;16:76–115.

Plasilova M, Stoilov I, Sarfarazi M, et al. Identification of a single ancestral CYP1B1 mutation in Slovak Gypsies (Roms) affected with primary congenital glaucoma. *J Med Genet.* 1999;36:290–294.

Taylor RH, Ainsworth JR, Evans AR, et al. The epidemiology of pediatric glaucoma: the Toronto experience. *J AAPOS.* 1999;3:308–315.

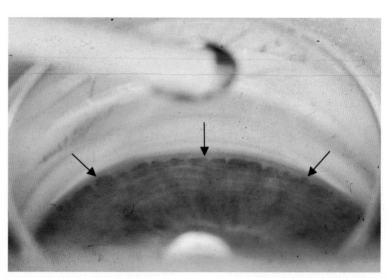

FIGURE 3-1. Gonioscopic view of a child with infantile glaucoma angle showing patches of high iris insertion (*arrows*).

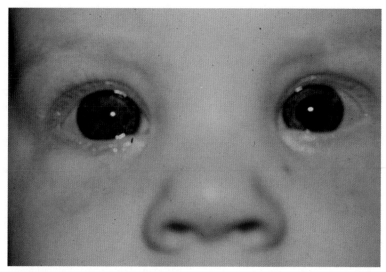

FIGURE 3-2. Buphthalmos and corneal clouding of the right eye. Miosis in the right eye is caused by the use of pilocarpine.

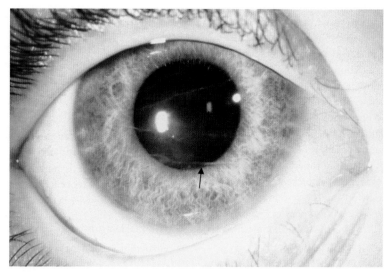

FIGURE 3-3. Haab striae, which are breaks in Descemet's membrane, are delineated by the appearance of two scrolled back edges (*arrows* denote the bottom Haab stria; there is also one more superiorly).

JUVENILE OPEN-ANGLE GLAUCOMA

Juvenile open-angle glaucoma (JOAG) is a form of open-angle primary glaucoma unassociated with ocular malformations, with an age of onset from age 4 to 40 years old. JOAG generally has a more aggressive course than the later onset adult primary open-angle glaucoma.

Epidemiology and Etiology

• The incidence of JOAG is 1 per 50,000 cases of all glaucoma. It has autosomal dominant inheritance with variable expression and penetrance. The most commonly mutated gene is the myocilin gene (*MYOC*) on chromosome 1q21-q31 (termed GLC1A). Myocilin is a glycoprotein that is expressed in the trabecular meshwork, with its function unknown. Mutations in the *CYP1B1* gene on chromosome 2p21 have been associated with autosomal recessive inheritance of juvenile onset glaucoma. Patients with a mutation in *CYP1B1* in addition to *MYOC* have a more severe phenotype than those with *MYOC* mutation alone. The pathophysiology of JOAG is unknown but is thought to be impaired aqueous outflow through the trabecular meshwork. There are usually no abnormalities on gonioscopy in affected patients, although there are histologic reports of thickening of the trabecular meshwork outflow system and clinical reports of increased iris processes ("pectinate ligaments") crossing the trabecular meshwork.

• Genetic studies of large families (e.g., the one shown in .2) demonstrated that defects or mutations in the myocilin gene are a cause of JOAG. Most cases of JOAG that have a strong family history of disease are associated with defects in the myocilin gene (*MYOC*). *Myocilin* associated glaucoma is inherited as an autosomal dominant trait. That is, patients carrying a *myocilin* mutation that causes JOAG have a 50% chance of passing the gene (and high risk for glaucoma) to their children. Several specific defects or mutations in *MYOC* that cause JOAG have been identified. Some patients have the typical clinical features of JOAG but do not have a family history of disease. *MYOC* has a less important role in these sporadic cases of JOAG.

History

• Patients are usually asymptomatic. Often, the disorder is noted as an incidental finding during routine examination.

• Because it is most commonly an autosomal dominant disorder, all family members of affected individuals should have a comprehensive examination.

Signs

• Complete anterior segment examination is important to assess for secondary causes of glaucoma. IOP measurement with routine ophthalmic examinations helps in identifying new cases.

• At-risk patients should be examined at least twice yearly.

• Patients with increased cup-to-disc ratio or asymmetry should undergo IOP measurements, gonioscopy, pachymetry, visual field testing, optical coherence tomography, and optic nerve photos with serial follow-up.

Differential Diagnosis

• Glaucoma secondary to uveitis

• Glaucoma associated with anterior segment dysgenesis

• Steroid-induced glaucoma

• Traumatic (e.g., angle recession) glaucoma

• Physiologic cupping

Diagnostic Evaluation

- At-risk children based on family history (one affected parent or sibling) should have IOP measurements serially even if sedation or anesthesia is required. Evaluation should include a comprehensive ophthalmic examination, including, vision, refraction, slit-lamp examination, pachymetry, gonioscopy, and ophthalmoscopy. Gonioscopy is not diagnostic but is useful in evaluating for secondary causes of glaucoma. The presence of increased numbers of iris processes may or may not represent an indicator of risk for JOAG.

- Patients with the clinical appearance of glaucomatous optic neuropathy with normal IOP on isolated visits should also undergo diurnal curve testing to assess pressure variation as well as maximum daily pressure.

- Automated visual field testing in young patients can be difficult, with Goldman visual field testing often being a better assessment tool.

- Optical coherence tomography currently has limited available normative data for children, but asymmetry between the two eyes and changes over time can be used as indicators of abnormality. Optic nerve photography is useful in documenting and monitoring change in the appearance of the optic nerves.

- Physiologic cupping, also an autosomal dominant condition, must be considered (Fig. 3-4) but is difficult to distinguish from JOAG other than the absence of elevated IOP, change over time, or visual field deficits. Physiologic cups tend to have very distinct sharp borders and may be eccentric within the disc. Patients' parents should be examined for similar findings and, if present, their IOP should be checked as well. It may take several visits over months or years to be confident that there is no progression and thus no JOAG.

Treatment and Prognosis

- JOAG tends to be more aggressive, more resistant to medical therapy, and associated with more severe visual impairment.

- The use of topical antiglaucoma medications is the first line of treatment followed by oral carbonic anhydrase inhibitors.

- JOAG patients require close follow-up until maintenance of an acceptable IOP is achieved.

- Most cases over the long term are progressive and require surgical intervention.

- Some evidence indicates that goniotomy and trabeculotomy can be successful. More traditionally, trabeculectomy or glaucoma drainage device surgery is the first surgical intervention. Trabeculectomy has similar success rates to those done on patients with primary open-angle glaucoma.

REFERENCES

Jacobi PC, Dietlein TS, Krieglstein GK. Primary trabeculectomy in young adults: long-term clinical results and factors influencing the outcome. *Ophthalmic Surg Lasers.* 1999;30:637–646.

Park SC, Kee C. Large diurnal variation of intraocular pressure despite maximal medical treatment in juvenile open angle glaucoma. *J Glaucoma.* 2007;16:164–168.

Stoilova D, Child A, Brice G, et al. Novel TIGR/MYOC mutations in families with juvenile onset primary open angle glaucoma. *J Med Genet.* 1998;35:989–992.

Vincent AL, Billingsley G, Buys Y, et al. Digenic inheritance of early-onset glaucoma: CYP1B1, a potential modifier gene. *Am J Hum Genet.* 2002;70:448–460.

Yeung HH, Walton DS. Goniotomy for juvenile open-angle glaucoma. *J Glaucoma.* 2010;19:1–4.

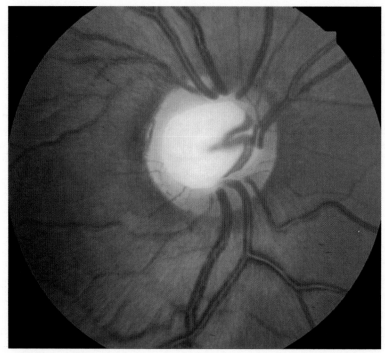

FIGURE 3-4. Physiologic cup. Note the sharp margin to the cup and scooped-out appearance. The vessels disappear as they turn posteriorly at the margin of the cup. The father, who did not have glaucoma, has a similar appearance to his optic nerve heads.

APHAKIC GLAUCOMA

Aphakic glaucoma is glaucoma that develops in an eye that is aphakic.

Epidemiology and Etiology

• Aphakic glaucoma is the most common complication of congenital cataract surgery with an incidence up to 32%. Theories as to the etiology include abnormal development of the anterior chamber angle, genetic predisposition, barotrauma incurred during surgery, decreased structural support to the drainage angle from aphakia, vitreous affecting angle structures, and release of chemical mediators that affect aqueous drainage.

• Despite advances in cataract surgery, it is clear that the prevention of glaucoma after cataract surgery has not been well understood. Even with the use of intraocular lens implantation in the pediatric population, the incidence of glaucoma appears to be unchanged.

• Factors associated with a higher risk of development of glaucoma are surgery within the first year of life, corneal diameter less than 10 mm, presence of other ocular anomalies, retained lens material, nuclear cataract, and eyes that require secondary surgeries.

History

• Similar to congenital infantile glaucoma, the symptom triad of photophobia, epiphora, and blepharospasm is often seen in those who develop aphakic glaucoma before age 3 years.

• Most patients are asymptomatic.

• The onset of glaucoma may occur early after surgery or later in childhood, with the average age to onset approximately 4 to 8 years after surgery.

• Routine lifelong screening of all aphakic patients is important for the early diagnosis of glaucoma.

Signs

• Early signs of glaucoma include a decrease in the amount of aphakic refraction (rapid loss of hyperopia caused by globe elongation), corneal clouding, and increased corneal diameter in patients who develop glaucoma generally before age 3 years old.

• Most patients are asymptomatic, and elevated IOP and optic nerve cupping are found on screening examination.

Differential Diagnosis

• Primary infantile glaucoma

• Anterior segment dysgenesis

• Uveitic glaucoma

• Traumatic glaucoma

Diagnostic Evaluation

• Pediatric patients who are left aphakic after cataract surgery should be examined for glaucoma on a regular basis, certainly no less than annually. When patients are too young for IOP measurement or optic nerve evaluation, an examination under anesthesia or sedation may be needed.

• Early signs of glaucoma include a decrease in the amount of aphakic refraction, corneal clouding, increased corneal diameter in young patients, and optic nerve cupping. The presence of peripheral or midperipheral anterior synechia or posterior synechia with iris bombe speaks to an inflammatory component.

• Biomicroscopy, corneal diameter measurement, pachymetry (which is often elevated in aphakia and pseudophakia), gonioscopy, axial length measurement, and optic nerve photography are all important components of an examination under anesthesia.

• Gonioscopy may show an angle configuration similar to that seen in primary infantile glaucoma (Fig. 3-5) or may have peripheral anterior synechia.

- Preoperative evaluation and measurements are useful in monitoring progression in those who require cataract surgery if aphakic or pseudophakic glaucoma later develops.

Treatment and Prognosis

- The first line of treatment of patients with aphakic glaucoma is one or more antiglaucoma medications, which in many cases prove effective in lowering the IOP.

- When topical and oral medications fail, surgery is often successful, with goniotomy or trabeculotomy surgery being effective in approximately 55% of patients.

- If the above procedures fail, then a trabeculectomy or glaucoma drainage device may be implanted. Endoscopic diode cyclophotoabaltion may provide another early option for treatment. Otherwise, cycloablation plays a role in cases of refractive glaucoma.

- Early detection and treatment of glaucoma are important in improving the likelihood of preventing optic nerve progression and preserving visual function.

- Aggressive treatment of refractive error, amblyopia, and visually significant optical opacities are also vital components of pediatric patients' eye care.

REFERENCES

Bothun ED, Guo Y, Christiansen SP, et al. Outcome of angle surgery in children with aphakic glaucoma. *J AAPOS.* 2010;14:235–239.

Chen TC, Walton DS, Bhatia LS. Aphakic glaucoma after congenital cataract surgery. *Arch Ophthalmol.* 2004; 122:1819–1825.

Levin AV. Aphakic glaucoma: a never-ending story? *Br J Ophthalmol.* 2007;91:1574–1575.

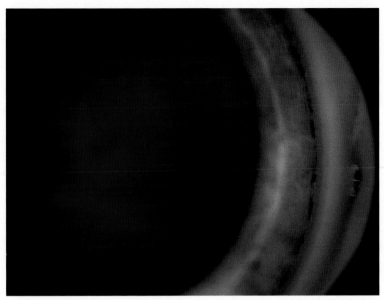

FIGURE 3-5. Gonioscopy of the angle in aphakic glaucoma appears similar to infantile glaucoma with patches of high iris insertion. This patient may be a good candidate for goniolytic surgery.

UVEITIC GLAUCOMA

The term *uveitic glaucoma* describes glaucoma that results as a complication of uveitis.

Epidemiology and Etiology

- The prevalence of pediatric uveitis is 30 cases per 100,000. Over a 5-year follow-up period, 35% of all children with uveitis had an episode of elevated IOP.

- Uveitis is associated with an increased risk of glaucoma not only because of the underlying process of uveitis but also because of the long-term use of corticosteroid treatments.

- The pathophysiology of uveitis inducing glaucoma is complex. In uveitis, vascular permeability is increased in the ciliary body, which results in aqueous hypersecretion and increased protein content. There is an increase in aqueous prostaglandins, which increases uveoscleral outflow at low concentrations but decreases uveoscleral outflow at higher concentrations.

- Aqueous outflow through the trabecular meshwork can be decreased by inflammatory cells and fibrin in the angle. Uveitis may also induce swelling or dysfunction of the trabecular meshwork and trabecular endothelium, decreasing outflow (trabeculitis).

- Peripheral anterior synechiae form in uveitis, with the most severe cases resulting in angle-closure glaucoma.

- Posterior synechia can result in pupillary block with iris bombe (see Fig. 3-6).

- Chronic inflammation and ischemia can lead to neovascular glaucoma.

- Although glaucoma can occur in every type of uveitis, certain etiologies of uveitis have a higher incidence, particularly juvenile idiopathic arthritis (JIA) at 16%.

History

- Acute anterior uveitis is characterized by photophobia, pain, redness, decreased vision, and epiphora.

- In posterior uveitis, the only symptoms may be floaters and blurred vision.

- Children with JIA are usually asymptomatic with regards to ocular involvement until late in the disease when they may present with irregularity of the pupil, whitening of the cornea from band keratopathy or decreased vision from cataracts, inflammation, and posterior synechiae.

- Glaucoma is asymptomatic unless an acute significant elevation in IOP occurs.

Signs

- In patients with uveitis, it is important to obtain a thorough history, including past medical history and review of symptoms.

- Slit-lamp examination is useful to quantify the amount of inflammation, assess peripheral and central anterior chamber depth, and assess the presence of posterior synechiae and neovascularization.

- Peripheral anterior synechiae form across the angle and are visualized on gonioscopy.

- The extent of peripheral anterior synechiae is not diagnostic for glaucoma but is a risk factor.

- As in all forms of glaucoma, optic nerve evaluation is important in diagnosing and monitoring disease progression.

- Secondary diagnostic tests such as optical coherence tomography and visual fields become more difficult because media opacities are more likely to be present in patients with uveitis.

- Despite active or inactive disease, continued monitoring for glaucoma is imperative.

Differential Diagnosis

- Steroid-induced glaucoma
- Angle-closure glaucoma
- Axenfeld Rieger spectrum
- Tumor (masquerade syndrome, e.g., leukemia, retinoblastoma)
- Ghost cell glaucoma
- Traumatic glaucoma

Diagnostic Evaluation

- As in all cases of uveitis, the extent of ocular involvement is determined by a comprehensive ophthalmic examination.
- A thorough history is obtained, including current complaints, medications, past medical history, and a review of systems.
- On slit-lamp biomicroscopy, the examination of the anterior segment includes cornea for keratic precipitates, band keratopathy and epithelial dendrites, anterior chamber depth, and evaluation for cells and flare; examination of the iris for stromal atrophy, iris nodules, posterior synechiae, and peripheral anterior synechiae; and examination of the lens for cataract.
- IOP should be checked on all patients with uveitis during virtually every visit.
- Shallowing of the anterior chamber, increased IOP, and peripheral anterior synechiae are indications for performing gonioscopy.
- Dilation with thorough examination of the posterior segment is necessary to help determine the extent as well as the cause of the uveitis. The optic nerve appearance should also be monitored for changes of glaucomatous optic neuropathy.
- In patients with acute uveitis and healthy optic nerves, the transient elevated IOP can be monitored because a decrease may occur with aggressive treatment of the inflammation. Chronic and recurrent uveitis with elevated IOP or at-risk nerves requires a lower threshold for treatment.

- A steroid-related increase in IOP rarely occurs within 2 weeks of initiating treatment, but the clearance of protein and cells from the anterior chamber may cause an acute and often transient elevation of IOP.
- The distinction between steroid responsiveness versus uveitic glaucoma may be achieved by changing treatment to a non-glaucomagenic anti-inflammatory agent (e.g., fluorometholone) or steroid-sparing systemic agents (e.g., methotrexate, anti–tumor necrosis factor [TNF] agents) without starting glaucoma drops.
- If the uveitis cannot be managed without continuing steroid therapy, then medical and, as needed, surgical glaucoma management are required.

Treatment and Prognosis

- The prognosis of uveitic glaucoma depends on the underlying disease and success of the treatment regimen.
- Treatment includes treating the underlying disease, ocular inflammation, and glaucoma.
- Oral immunomodulatory medications may be necessary to provide control of the underlying disease. In patients with JIA, use of systemic anti-TNF agents is thought to lower the ocular complications of cataracts, band keratopathy, and glaucoma.
- Control of chronic uveitis, especially in JIA, may require chronic frequent topical steroids with slow weans over months to years.
- Mydriatic drops are essential in decreasing the risk of pupillary block by increasing the pupil size and breaking posterior synechiae.
- Elevated IOP is treated by determining the glaucoma mechanism (e.g., steroid-induced vs. iris bombe).

- Patients with glaucoma are treated primarily with topical antiglaucoma drops. The general rule is that surgery is to be avoided when possible because the eyes have an aggressive inflammatory response.

- Patients who do require surgery should be treated with preoperative oral prednisone as well as frequent topical prednisone.

- Goniotomy represents an effective first-line surgical option for young patients with chronic uveitis and glaucoma without significant peripheral anterior synechia or iris bombe.

- Trabeculectomy, especially in pediatric patients with uveitis, has a lower success rate because of aggressive scar formation.

- Glaucoma drainage devices are used in refractory cases and can provide good long-term glaucoma control comparable to those without uveitis.

- Intraocular lens implantation in children with uveitic cataracts may cause significant aggravation of the iritis and induce or worsen uveitis.

REFERENCES

Freedman SF, Rodriguez-Rosa RE, Rojas MC, et al. Goniotomy for glaucoma secondary to chronic childhood uveitis. *Am J Ophthalmol.* 2002;133:617–621.

Rachmiel R, Trope GE, Buys YM, et al. Ahmed glaucoma valve implantation in uveitic glaucoma versus open-angle glaucoma patients. *Can J Ophthalmol.* 2008;43:462-467.

Sijssens KM, Rothova A, Berendschot TT, et al. Ocular hypertension and secondary glaucoma in children with uveitis. *Ophthalmology.* 2006;113:853–859 e852.

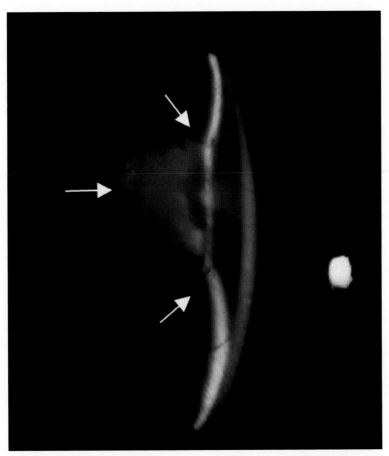

FIGURE 3-6. A patient with juvenile idiopathic arthritis and 360 degrees of posterior synechiae (*arrows*) leading to iris bombe. The anterior chamber is deep centrally and shallow peripherally. The patient also has a total white cataract.

STURGE-WEBER SYNDROME

Encephalotrigeminal angiomatosis (Sturge-Weber syndrome) is a nonheritable syndrome of port wine mark; ipsilateral risk of glaucoma; and central nervous system (CNS) involvement, including possible developmental delay, seizures, and radiographic evidence of leptomeningeal calcification or cerebral atrophy.

Epidemiology and Etiology

- There is no gender, race, or sexual predilection to the disorder.

- The classic Sturge-Weber port wine mark respects the midline and follows the distribution of the trigeminal ganglion branches (Fig. 3-7).

- Up to one-third of patients develop glaucoma on the ipsilateral side, and eyes at higher risk have the upper eyelid affected.

- Whereas an onset of glaucoma early in life is thought to be the result of a developmental anomaly of the angle, later onset glaucoma, usually between 4 and 40 years old, is related to elevated episcleral venous pressure.

History

- The facial cutaneous lesion is usually the first component of Sturge-Weber syndrome to be observed and is visible at birth. It may become darker with age and is more noticeable in those with fair skin.

- Patients with a port wine mark of the face involving any portion of the eyelids require referral for a complete ophthalmic evaluation with screening for glaucoma.

- Early-onset glaucoma presents with buphthalmos, epiphora, and photophobia as in primary infantile glaucoma.

- Later-onset glaucoma is diagnosed based on screening ophthalmic examination because there are usually no symptoms.

Signs

- The port wine mark is a clinical marker to identify patients and eyes at risk for ocular complications.

- The hypervascularity of this disorder is evident on ocular examination with increased conjunctival and episcleral vascularity (Fig. 3-8) in up to 70% of patients.

- Heterochromia of the iris occurs in 10%, with increased pigment on the affected side caused by a relative increase in melanocyte activity.

- Approximately 10% of patients with Sturge-Weber syndrome have bilateral disease.

- Diffuse choroidal hemangioma is based on tumor appearance with indirect ophthalmoscopy with indistinguishable choroidal markings (Fig. 3-9). It is usually seen in the posterior pole and can show thickening and elevation during adolescence and adulthood.

- Secondary changes to the overlying retina include vascular tortuosity, exudate, cystic changes, gliosis, and edema.

- The risk for glaucoma is increased when choroidal hemangioma is present.

- Clinical signs in infants and toddlers are similar to those seen in primary infantile glaucoma.

- On gonioscopy, blood visualized in Schlemm's canal is suggestive of elevated episcleral venous pressure.

Differential Diagnosis

- Capillary hemangioma
- Klippel-Trenaunay-Weber syndrome (Sturge-Weber syndrome plus hemihypertrophy of soft and bony tissues)
- Transient nevus flammeus of infancy
- Primary infantile glaucoma

- Primary JOAG
- Cutis marmorata telangiectasia congenita
- Phakomatosis pigmentovascularis

Diagnostic Evaluation

- Ocular testing for glaucoma includes a careful assessment of IOP, corneal diameter, pachymetry (often elevated in those with Sturge-Weber syndrome), gonioscopy, cycloplegic refraction, axial length, and optic nerve cupping evaluation.
- Ocular ultrasonography may be useful showing high internal reflectivity in a solid echogenic mass characteristic of choroidal hemangiomas.
- CT and MRI can be used to detect malformations in the CNS.

Treatment and Prognosis

- Topical antiglaucoma medications are the initial treatment modality except in infancy when the treatment paradigm is usually surgical (goniotomy or trabeculotomy) as for primary infantile glaucoma.

- As the underlying pathophysiology becomes elevated episcleral venous pressure, medical treatment is still the desired first-line option, but trabeculectomy or drainage tube surgery may be needed.
- There is an increased risk of choroidal effusion and hemorrhage secondary to surgery.
- A diffuse choroidal hemangioma is associated with an increased risk of nonrhegmatogenous retinal detachment as well as vision loss caused by cystoid macular edema.
- Photocoagulation with or without pars plana vitrectomy and drainage of the subretinal fluid have met with limited success and are usually reserved for those patients with central vision loss caused by the hemangioma.

REFERENCES

Aggarwal NK, Gandham SB, Weinstein R, et al. Heterochromia iridis and pertinent clinical findings in patients with glaucoma associated with Sturge-Weber syndrome. *J Pediatr Ophthalmol Strabismus.* 2010;47:361–365.

Sullivan TJ, Clarke MP, Morin JD. The ocular manifestations of the Sturge-Weber syndrome. *J Pediatr Ophthalmol Strabismus.* 1992;29:349–356.

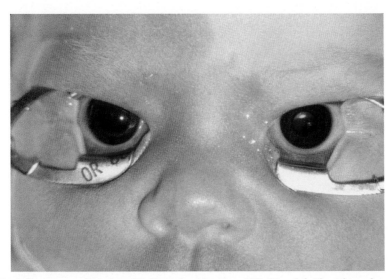

FIGURE 3-7. Port wine mark involving V1–V3 on the right side and V2–V3 on left. The right eye has buphthalmos with corneal clouding.

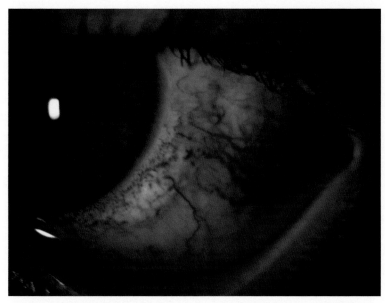

FIGURE 3-8. Dilated tortuous conjunctival and episcleral vessels, ipsilateral to the side with port wine mark (not shown). (Courtesy Rachel Sobel, MD, Wills Eye Institute, Philadelphia.)

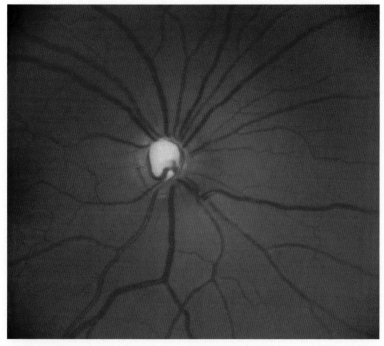

FIGURE 3-9. Choroidal hemangioma. Note the absence of choroidal markings and diffuse red-orange hue. Note the increased cup-to-disc ratio caused by glaucoma and the choroidal hemangioma.

CONGENITAL ECTROPION UVEAE

Congenital ectropion uveae is a rare disorder characterized by persistent cells of neural crest origin on the anterior surface of the iris and trabecular meshwork associated with varying degrees of ectropion uvea. Patients have an anterior insertion of the iris and dysgenesis of the anterior segment angle with an increased risk of glaucoma.

Epidemiology and Etiology

- Congenital ectropion uveae is a rare condition with an undefined incidence. It is a unilateral developmental disorder that involves the iris and anterior chamber angle, resulting from a neural crest migration abnormality.

- Histopathologic studies have also described a fibrovascular surface membrane covering the anterior iris surface, suggesting that contraction causes the ectropion uveae and further growth into the angle inducing glaucoma.

- No genetic etiology or heritability has been described.

History

- Patients are usually asymptomatic. Often, the disorder is noted as an incidental finding during routine pediatric or ophthalmic examination. It may present with a parental concern of pupillary asymmetry with the ectropion uvea, creating the illusion of a bigger pupil.

Signs

- Slit-lamp biomicroscopy reveals iris pigment epithelium on the anterior surface of the iris (Fig. 3-10). The remainder of the iris appears smooth and cryptless with an overlying whitish coating.

- On gonioscopy, there is anterior insertion of the iris onto the trabecular meshwork and goniodysgenesis. IOP elevation and optic nerve cupping are indicative of the development of glaucoma.

- Mild ptosis with good levator function is reported in up to 50% of cases.

Differential Diagnosis

- Axenfeld-Rieger spectrum
- Anisocoria
- Iridocorneal endothelial syndrome
- Uveitis
- Rubeosis
- Trauma

Diagnostic Evaluation

- Congenital ectropion uveae can be associated with other anterior segment anomalies; thus, a thorough ophthalmoscopic and systemic evaluation is indicated.

- Reported rare associations include neurofibromatosis, facial hemihypertrophy, Axenfeld-Rieger spectrum, and Prader-Willi syndrome.

Treatment and Prognosis

- Although the actual anomaly of ectropion uveae is considered nonprogressive, this disorder is an indication for screening and continued surveillance for the development of glaucoma.

- Glaucoma almost inevitably develops with the age of onset ranging from early childhood to adulthood.

- Treatment with standard antiglaucoma medications can result in an initial IOP-lowering effect but is short lived, and definitive treatment of filtering or tube surgery is required.

REFERENCES

Dowling JL Jr, Albert DM, Nelson LB, et al. Primary glaucoma associated with iridotrabecular dysgenesis and ectropion uveae. *Ophthalmology.* 1985;92: 912–921.

Harasymowycz PJ, Papamatheakis DG, Eagle RC Jr, et al. Congenital ectropion uveae and glaucoma. *Arch Ophthalmol.* 2006;124:271–273.

Ritch R, Forbes M, Hetherington J Jr, et al. Congenital ectropion uveae with glaucoma. *Ophthalmology.* 1984; 91:326–331.

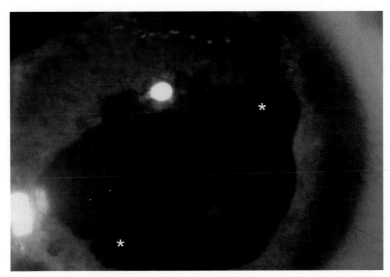

FIGURE 3-10. Iris pigment epithelium on the anterior surface of the iris (*asterisk*). Much of the remaining iris appears whitened with a loss of iris crypts.

ANIRIDIA

Aniridia is complete or partial iris hypoplasia with associated foveal hypoplasia, resulting in decreased visual acuity and early onset nystagmus. Aniridia occurs as a result of a sporadic or autosomal dominantly inherited mutation affecting *PAX6* gene expression.

Epidemiology and Etiology

- The incidence of aniridia is one in 40,000 to 100,000.

- Disease-causing mutations have been reported in the *PAX6* gene (11p13) or the upstream regulatory region controlling its expression. The *PAX6* gene encodes a transcriptional regulator that controls the expression of other genes involved in oculogenesis as well as other developmental processes.

- Up to 20% of sporadic cases of aniridia have been found to have a deletion in 11p13 on cytogenetic testing. This deletion may involve the Wilms' tumor gene (*WT1*) and intervening genes as part of WAGR syndrome (Wilms' tumor, aniridia, genital anomalies, and retardation).

- Patients with aniridia have up to a 50% lifetime risk of developing glaucoma.

History

- Aniridia is discovered early in life usually by the presence of nystagmus in infancy.

- Visual acuity, when able to be tested, is often in the range of 20/100 to 20/200 but may be as good as 20/40 in patients with low expression.

- Patients may also experience photophobia.

- Only 20% of affected patients have a positive family history.

Signs

- Aniridia shows variable expression regarding the extent of iris abnormality and other ocular findings. Foveal hypoplasia is the primary cause of the decreased vision and is evident on ophthalmoscopy and can be confirmed with optical coherence tomography.

- Other frequent ocular anomalies include corneal pannus, limbal stem cell deficiency, optic nerve hypoplasia, cataract (most commonly anterior pyramidal) and glaucoma.

- Less commonly, patients may have ectopia lentis, microphthalmia, and Peters' anomaly.

- Patients with aniridia and new-onset eye irritation require urgent evaluation for glaucoma as well as keratopathy. Aniridic keratopathy results from abnormal limbal stem cell development with fragility of the epithelial cells, poor wound healing, and reduced epithelial adhesion.

Differential Diagnosis

- Axenfeld-Rieger spectrum
- Iris coloboma
- Gillespie syndrome
- Trauma or iatrogenic iris defect
- Bilateral congenital mydriasis
- Pharmacologic mydriasis

Diagnostic Evaluation

- The presentation of aniridia can be variable ranging from enlarged nonreactive pupils to complete iris absence. The amount of residual iris may differ between the two eyes.

- Slit-lamp biomicroscopy is needed to detect corneal pannus, which often begins as peripheral grey superficial avascular changes.

- Examination under anesthesia is useful in obtaining a complete ophthalmic examination, including IOP measurement and gonioscopy in young infants. In young children, the development and progression of glaucoma can be assessed by an increase in corneal diameter, increase in the axial length, and loss of hyperopia or increased myopia on cycloplegic refraction.

- Gonioscopic examination reveals a rudimentary iris, rather than complete absence, with areas of upturned iris blocking the trabecular meshwork (**Fig. 3-11**). Glaucoma in aniridia is common and may be caused by primary goniodysgenesis, occlusion of the trabecular meshwork by the iris stub, or aplasia of Schlemm's canal.

- In infants with significant corneal opacities, an anterior segment ultrasound biomicroscopy can demonstrate iris hypoplasia and show angle anomalies.

- Systemic evaluation for associated findings with aniridia and WAGR includes cryptorchidism and other genitourinary abnormalities, intellectual disability, neurologic abnormalities (e.g., hypertonia, hypotonia, epilepsy), skeletal anomalies (craniofacial anomalies, growth retardation, or scoliosis), hearing loss, and obesity.

Treatment and Prognosis

- Individuals without a family history of aniridia should undergo cytogenetic and molecular genetic testing to detect possible WAGR syndrome. Those with aniridia and *WT1* mutation require renal ultrasound every 3 months until approximately 8 years old. In the absence of molecular testing to exclude WAGR, renal screening should be conducted every 6 months. Those without WAGR still require continued periodic ophthalmic examinations for glaucoma, corneal abnormalities, and cataracts.

- The treatment of glaucoma in aniridia is based on gonioscopy and age. Goniosurgery may be useful as a primary procedure, particularly in infants. The decision to perform cataract surgery requires consideration of other causes of diminished vision such foveal hypoplasia, optic nerve hypoplasia, and nystagmus. Aniridic eyes can have poor zonular stability, affecting how the surgery is done and the type of lens implant used.

REFERENCES

Ramaesh K, Ramaesh T, Dutton GN, et al. Evolving concepts on the pathogenic mechanisms of aniridia related keratopathy. *Int J Biochem Cell Biol.* 2005;37: 547–557.

Schneider S, Osher RH, Burk SE, et al. Thinning of the anterior capsule associated with congenital aniridia. *J Cataract Refract Surg.* 2003;29:523–525.

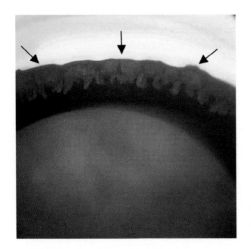

FIGURE 3-11. Gonioscopic view of aniridic eye with the iris root turned up in multiple places (*arrows*), obstructing the trabecular meshwork.

POSTERIOR EMBRYOTOXON

Posterior embryotoxon is the anterior displacement of Schwalbe's line and structurally represents an anteriorized junction of the peripheral termination of Descemet's membrane. Clinically, it appears as a white circumferential line on the inner surface of the cornea near the limbus.

Epidemiology and Etiology

● The prevalence of posterior embryotoxon is 6.8% to 32% of the general population. It may occur as an isolated finding or be associated with other anterior segment or systemic findings as in Axenfeld-Rieger spectrum and Alagille syndrome. It considered a developmental neuralcrestopathy.

● There has not been a specific mutated gene associated with isolated posterior embryotoxon, but mutations in *PITX2*, *FOXC1*, and *JAG1* each are associated with the clinical findings of the syndromic forms.

History

● Patients are usually asymptomatic. Often the disorder is noted as an incidental finding during slit-lamp biomicroscopy and gonioscopy.

Important Clinical Signs

● Posterior embryotoxon is visible with slit-lamp biomicroscopy as a fine silver-white circumferential line on the inner aspect of the cornea, anterior to the limbus (**Fig. 3-12**). It occurs more commonly nasally and temporally.

● The presence of iridocorneal strands to the posterior embryotoxon identifies the mildest form of the Axenfeld-Reiger spectrum. With the Axenfeld-Reiger spectrum, systemic anomalies include redundant periumbilical skin, abnormal facies, sensorineuronal hearing loss, skeletal malformations, and dental malformations.

● Ophthalmoscopic findings suggestive of Alagille syndrome include retinal pigment epithelial irregularities and optic nerve anomalies.

Differential Diagnosis

● Axenfeld-Rieger spectrum

● Alagille syndrome

● Peters' anomaly

● Cornea plana

● Mesodermal dysgenesis

● Peripheral anterior synechiae

● Haab stria

● Forceps injury

● Trauma

Diagnostic Evaluation

● The characteristic appearance of posterior embryotoxon should enable the clinician to make the diagnosis and differentiate it from other lesions. Gonioscopy can be used to identify cases that are not otherwise evident on slit-lamp examination.

● Although not needed to make the diagnosis, anterior segment optical coherence tomography can also show the abnormality. Histologically, it consists of collagen fibers covered by a thin layer of Descemet's membrane and endothelium.

● The risk of glaucoma in isolated posterior embryotoxon is not well defined but likely elevated. In Axenfeld-Rieger spectrum, the risk may be as high as 50%.

● Patients should have a complete ophthalmic examination, including IOP and dilated fundus examination. More aggressive monitoring is needed in patients with findings of Axenfeld-Rieger spectrum.

Treatment and Prognosis

- The extent of posterior embryotoxon is not predictive of the presence of an underlying condition. The finding should prompt further anterior segment examination, gonioscopy, and assessment for possible glaucoma as well as systemic examination for syndromic findings.

- Screening of family members may be helpfully clinically because presentation is variable.

REFERENCES

Ozeki H, Shirai S, Majima A, et al. Clinical evaluation of posterior embryotoxon in one institution. *Jpn J Ophthalmol.* 1997;41:422–425.

Rennie CA, Chowdhury S, Khan J, et al. The prevalence and associated features of posterior embryotoxon in the general ophthalmic clinic. *Eye (Lond).* 2005; 19:396–399.

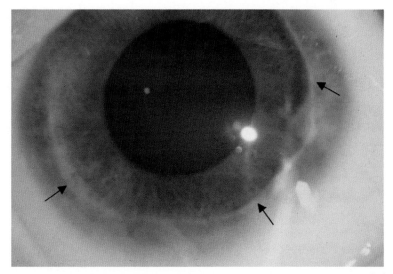

FIGURE 3-12. Posterior embryotoxon appears as a white or grey circumferential line anterior to the limbus (*arrows*).

Iris Anomalies

Michael J. Bartiss and Bruce M. Schall ■

CENTRAL PUPILLARY CYSTS (PUPILLARY MARGIN EPITHELIAL CYSTS)

Etiology

- Usually congenital in origin

- Can be acquired from cholinesterase inhibiting eye drops, such as phospholine iodide, when used in young, phakic patients to treat accommodative esotropia

- Rarely inherited

Symptoms

- Patients are usually asymptomatic.

- Pigmented epithelial cysts occurring at the pupillary border (Fig. 4-1)

- May be detected by pediatrician on red reflex testing of neonate

Signs

- Pigmented cysts along the margin of the pupil of involved eyes

- Have a nontransparent lining (as opposed to iris stromal cysts)

- Rarely increase in size and typically remain stationary

Differential Diagnosis

- Iris stromal cysts

- Ciliary body cysts

- Iris melanoma

Treatment

- Congenital pupillary margin epithelial cysts rarely require treatment; they usually remain stationary in size or slowly involute over time.

- If size and location cause visual compromise, surgical intervention may be indicated.

- Acquired pupillary margin cysts from cholinesterase-inhibiting eye drops can be prevented with the use of daily phenylephrine (2.5%) eyedrops.

Prognosis

- Excellent; rarely require treatment

- Complications can include formation of iris flocculi in cases of cyst rupture, glaucoma, and spontaneous intraocular detachment of the cysts.

- If treatment is required, can be treated with simple excision or yttrium aluminium garnet (YAG) puncture

REFERENCES

Shields JA, Kline MW, Augsburger JJ. Primary iris cysts: a review of the literature and report of 62 cases. *Br J Ophthalmol.* 1984;68(3):152–166.

Shields JA, Shields CL, Lois N, et al. Iris cysts in children: classification, incidence and management: the 1998 Torrence A Makley, Jr. lecture. *Br J Ophthalmol.* 1999;83(3):334–338.

Sidoti PA, Valencia M, Chen M. Echographic evaluation of primary cysts of the iris pigment epithelium. *Am J Ophthalmol.* 1995;120:161–167.

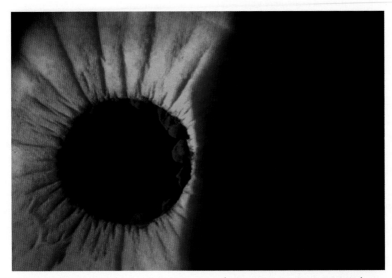

FIGURE 4-1. Pigmented cysts along the margin of the pupil. (Courtesy of Judith Lavrich, MD.)

ANIRIDIA

Etiology

- Bilateral disorder characterized by under-development (rather than true absence of the iris) with rudimentary iris located peripherally

- Associated with *PAX6* gene (control gene for eye morphogenesis) on chromosome 11p13: involving inability of single gene allele to activate transduction of developmental genes (haploinsufficiency)

- Often associated with foveal hypoplasia, nystagmus, glaucoma, optic nerve hypoplasia, cataracts, and acquired corneal pannus

- Autosomal dominant (complete penetrance with variable expressivity), autosomal recessive (Gillespie's syndrome with mental retardation and cerebellar ataxia), and sporadic inheritance patterns

- Two-thirds of children with aniridia have affected parents

- Sporadic aniridia is associated with an increased incidence of Wilms' tumor.

- WAGR complex (Wilms' tumor, aniridia, genitourinary malformations, and mental retardation) occurs from contiguous gene deletions.

Symptoms

- Clinical absence of the iris

- Subnormal visual acuity common (usually less than 20/100)

- Nystagmus

- Photophobia

Signs

- Apparent bilateral absence or severe hypoplasia of iris (**Fig. 4-2**)

- Congenital nystagmus

- Acquired corneal pannus

- Strabismus

- Cataract

- Ectopia lentis

- Glaucoma

- Posterior synechiae

Differential Diagnosis

- Other causes of pupillary dilation (e.g., pharmacologically dilated pupils, Aides pupil)

Treatment

- Evaluation with a geneticist

- Screening for Wilms' tumor includes abdominal ultrasonography evaluations every 3 months until age 7 to 8 years of age

- Screen for glaucoma and treat if present.

- Cataract surgery if visually significant cataract is present

- Maximize visual potential with appropriate refractive error correction.

- Polarized sun wear or use of Transitions spectacles lenses to decrease glare and photophobia

REFERENCES

Adeoti CO, Afolabi AA, Ashaye AO, et al. Bilateral sporadic aniridia: review of management. *Clin Ophthalmol.* 2010;4:1085–1089.

Lee H, Meyers K, Lanigan B, et al. Complications and visual prognosis in children with aniridia. *J Pediatr Ophthalmol Strabismus.* 2010;47(4):205–210.

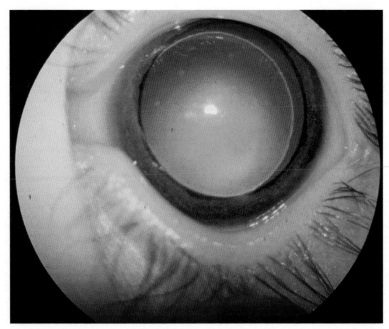

FIGURE 4-2. Severe hypoplasia of iris with outline of lens visible. (Courtesy of Alex V. Levin, MD, MHSc, Wills Eye Institute, Philadelphia.)

BRUSHFIELD SPOTS

Etiology

- Occur in up to 90% of patients with Down's syndrome (trisomy 21)
- Can be present in patients without Down's syndrome

Symptoms

- Patients are asymptomatic.

Signs

- Whitish elevated spots on the anterior surface of the iris, often occurring in a concentric ring around the pupil (Fig. 4-3)
- Congenital, normal, to hypercellular hypopigmented areas of iris tissue with surrounding relative stromal hypoplasia

Differential Diagnosis

- Wolfflin nodules (similar appearing nodules occurring in patients without Down's syndrome, which are accumulations of fibrous tissue in the anterior border layer of the iris)
- Iris nevi
- Brushfield's spots
- Juvenile xanthogranuloma (JXG)
- Iris mamillations

Treatment

- No treatment indicated

Prognosis

- No effect on visual function
- Severity of functional cognitive impairment of patients with trisomy 21 is extremely variable.

REFERENCES

Brooke Williams RD. Brushfield spots and Wolfflin nodules in the iris: an appraisal in handicapped children. *Dev Med Child Neurol.* 1981;23(5):646–649.

Shapiro BL. Down syndrome and associated congenital malformations [review]. *J Neural Transm Suppl.* 2003;(67):207–214.

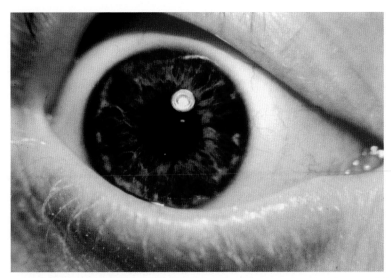

FIGURE 4-3. Hypopigmented elevated spots on the anterior iris surface in a concentric ring around the pupil. (Courtesy of Alex V. Levin, MD, MHSc, Wills Eye Institute, Philadelphia.)

ECOTOPIA LENTIS ET PUPILLAE

Etiology

- Autosomal recessive inherited, non-progressive disorder in which the pupil and lens are displaced in opposite directions (pupil usually inferonasally and lens superotemporally)
- Posterior displacement of lens–iris diaphragm
- Typically bilateral and asymmetric
- Believed to occur during neuroectodermal tissue development (pigmented layers of iris, iris dilator, and zonules are all involved)

Symptoms

- Decreased uncorrected visual acuity secondary dislocated lens

Signs

- Bilateral lens dislocation causing high myopia with astigmatism
- Asymmetrical, eccentrically located pupils (usually inferonasally)
- Slit-shaped or oval pupil (**Fig. 4-4A**)
- Persistent pupillary membrane is present in approximately 85% of affected individuals (**Fig. 4-4B**)
- Microspherophakia, miosis, and poor dilation with mydriatic agents
- Myopia, which may be severe
- May have an enlarged corneal diameter
- Cataract
- Abnormal iris transillumination
- Retinal detachment
- +/− Megalocornea

Differential Diagnosis

- Other causes for bilateral dislocated lenses, Marfan's syndrome, homocystinuria, Weil-Marchesani syndrome, sulfite oxidase deficiency, hyperlysinemia
- Iris coloboma
- Trauma to iris sphincter
- After anterior segment surgery
- Corectopia
- Axenfeld-Rieger syndrome

Treatment

- Refractive error correction to maximize visual potential
- Anisometropic amblyopia often occurs in the more affected eye. Amblyopia should be treated with correction of refractive and occlusion of fellow eye.
- May develop a visually significant cataract and therefore may require cataract surgery
- Screen for glaucoma.

Prognosis

- Nonprogressive; visual prognosis depends on timely treatment of refractive error. Amblyopia in more affected eye is often severe and may not respond to treatment.

REFERENCES

Byles DB, Nischal KK, Cheng H. Ectopia lentis et pupillae. A hypothesis revisited. *Ophthalmology.* 1998;105(7):1331–1336.

Colley A, Lloyd IC, Ridgway A, et al. Ectopia lentis et pupillae: the genetic aspects and differential diagnosis. *J Med Genet.* 1991;28(11):791–794.

Goldberg MF. Clinical manifestations of ectopia lentis et pupillae in 16 patients. *Ophthalmology.* 1988; 95(8):1080–1087.

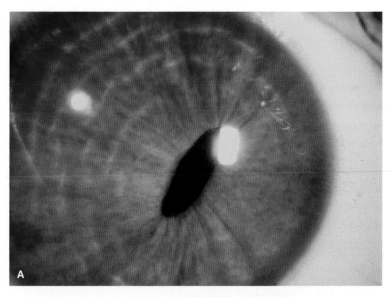

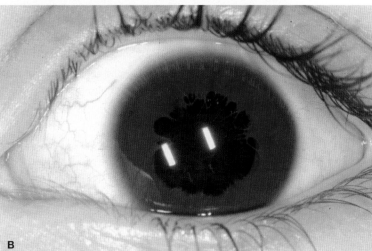

FIGURE 4-4. **A.** Inferonasally eccentrically located slit-shaped pupil. (Courtesy of Alex V. Levin, MD, MHSc, Wills Eye Institute, Philadelphia.) **B.** Note the persistent pupillary membrane, which is being stretched in this pharmacologically dilated pupil. The superior edge of the dislocated lens is visible.

HETEROCHROMIA IRIDIS

Etiology

- A congenital or acquired condition characterized by a relative hyperpigmentation or hypopigmentation of the involved iris

- Acquired cases of hyperpigmented irides in children include trauma, siderosis, iris ectropion syndrome, chronic iridocyclitis, and extensive rubeosis as well as intraocular surgery and topical prostaglandin analogue medications

- Ocular melanocytosis or oculodermal melanocytosis and sector iris hamartoma can also cause hyperpigmented irides.

- Congenital and acquired hypopigmented irides can occur because of Horner's syndrome, Fuchs heterochromia, Waardenburg-Klein syndrome, nonpigmented iris tumors, and hypomelanosis of Ito.

Symptoms

- Patients are typically asymptomatic in the absence of rubeosis, increased intraocular pressure (IOP), and intraocular inflammation.

Signs

- Different-colored irides with or without anatomical iris abnormalities

- In cases of melanosis oculi, the more pigmented iris may appear thicker with mamillations (Fig. 4-5).

- Associated with miosis and ptosis (typically 2 mm) on the ipsilateral side in cases of Horner's syndrome (Fig. 4-6)

Differential Diagnosis

- Differential diagnosis is extensive.

- Acquired cases of hyperpigmented irides in children include trauma, siderosis, iris ectropion syndrome, chronic iridocyclitis, and extensive rubeosis as well as intraocular surgery and topical prostaglandin analog medications.

- Ocular melanocytosis or oculodermal melanocytosis and sector iris hamartoma can also cause hyperpigmented irides.

- Congenital and acquired hypopigmented irides can occur because of Horner's syndrome, Fuchs heterochromia, Waardenburg-Klein syndrome, nonpigmented iris tumors, and hypomelanosis of Ito.

- Neuroblastoma (located along the sympathetic chain) must be ruled out in cases of Horner's syndrome, especially in acquired cases in children.

Treatment

- Assessment as to which iris has the abnormal color can often be assisted by assessing skin pigmentation, parental eye color, and earlier photographs of the patient.

- Timely and appropriate workup of acquired Horner's syndrome

- Hearing testing if Waardenburg's syndrome is suspected

- In cases of acquired hyperpigmentation, imaging may be needed to rule out an intraocular foreign body (siderosis) and intraocular tumor.

Prognosis

- Depends on the underlying cause

REFERENCES

Brazel SM, Sullivan TJ, Thorner PS, et al. Iris sector heterochromia as a marker for neural crest disease. *Arch Ophthalmol.* 1992;110(2):233–235.

Liu XZ, Newton VE, Read AP. Waardenburg syndrome type II: phenotypic findings and diagnostic criteria. *Am J Med Genet.* 1995 2;55(1):95–100.

Milunsky JM. Waardenburg syndrome type I. In: Pagon RA, Bird TC, Dolan CR, Stephens K, eds. *GeneReviews.* Seattle: University of Washington; 2004.

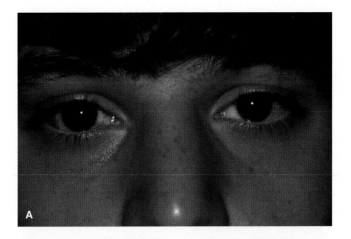

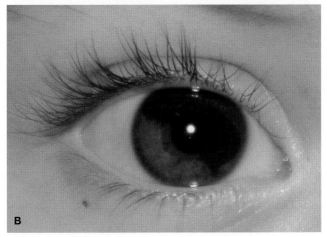

FIGURE 4-5. **A.** Right iris is more heavily pigmented in this child with melanosis oculi. **B.** Sector melanosis oculi.

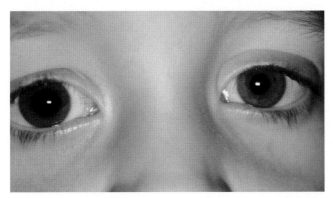

FIGURE 4-6. Left congenital Horner's syndrome. Note the miotic pupil, mild ptosis, and hypopigmented iris on the left. The ptosis is best observed by looking at the distance from the corneal light reflex to the pupillary margin.

IRIS COLOBOMA

Etiology

- Typically bilateral inferonasal defect in the iris caused by failure of embryonic fissure closure during the fifth gestation week

- May be part of a spectrum of anatomical developmental abnormalities including microphthalmia

- Autosomal dominant inheritance in approximately 20% of cases

- Atypical iris colobomas located other than inferonasally can occur and are probably caused by developmental abnormalities of the anterior hyaloids and papillary membrane systems and are not associated with posterior segment colobomas

- Numerous chromosomal abnormalities, including trisomy 13, 4p-, 11q- 13r, and 18r, are associated with colobomas.

- Numerous syndromes are associated with uveal colobomas, most notably CHARGE syndrome (coloboma of the eye or central nervous system anomalies, heart defects, atresia of the choanae, retardation of growth or development, genital or urinary defects, and ear anomalies or deafness).

- Other associated syndromes include Golz focal dermal hypoplasia, basal cell nevus syndrome, linear sebaceous syndrome, Klinefelter's syndrome, and Goldenhar's syndrome.

Symptoms

- Keyhole- or bulb-shaped pupil

- Patients are often asymptomatic if only the iris is involved.

- Patients are sometimes bothered by their cosmetic appearance.

- Visual acuity depends on involvement of the posterior segment.

Signs

- Inferonasal, lightbulb-shaped iris defect (Fig. 4-7)

- Colobomatous defect can also involve ciliary body, retina, choroid, and optic nerve. Lens zonules may be missing in a sector of the coloboma.

- Involvement may be asymmetric.

- Nystagmus presents in cases with concomitant bilateral optic nerve or macula involvement.

Differential Diagnosis

- Traumatic iris injury

- After an iridectomy

- Ectopic pupil

- Corectopia

Treatment

- Evaluation by a geneticist if other congenital anomalies are found or a syndrome is suspected

- Maximize visual acuity with appropriate refractive error correction.

- Colored contact lenses (with iris detail) are often helpful if psychosocial issues are present, especially in patients with lightly colored irides.

- Impact-resistant spectacles, especially in cases with functional vision in only one eye

Prognosis

- Visual prognosis depends on involvement of the optic disc and macula. Visual potential is very difficult to predict on the basis of clinical examination alone even in cases with significant posterior segment involvement.

- Visual acuity often remains stable after it has been maximized.

- Risk of retinal detachment

REFERENCES

Mets MB, Erzurum SA. Uveal tract in infants. In: Isenberg SJ, ed. *The Eye in Infancy.* 2nd ed. St. Louis: Mosby; 1994:308–317.

Onwochei BC, Simon JW, Bateman JB, et al. Ocular colobomata. *Survey Ophthalmol.* 2000;45:175–194.

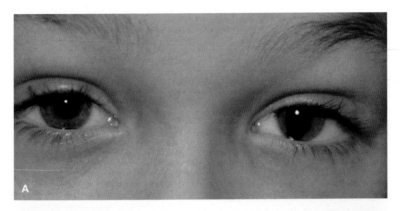

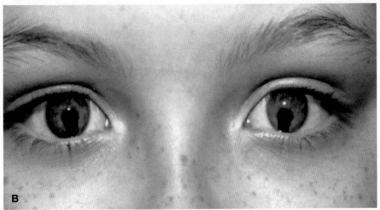

FIGURE 4-7. **A.** Unilateral iris coloboma. Lightbulb-shaped inferonasal defect in iris left eye. **B.** Bilateral iris coloboma.

IRIS STROMAL CYSTS

Etiology

- Probably occur because of sequestration of epithelial cells during embryologic development

- Typically contain goblet cells

Symptoms

- Can enlarge over time, obstructing the visual axis and causing decreased visual acuity

- Iritis with increased IOP and photophobia can occur if cysts leak.

- Often diagnosed during infancy

Signs

- Clear to whitish appearing cyst on anterior surface of the iris (Fig. 4-8)

- Epithelium-lined cysts occurring on the anterior surface of the iris with a visible vasculature

- May enlarge, causing decreased vision by obstructing the visual axis, iritis (from cyst leakage), corneal decompensation, and glaucoma

Differential Diagnosis

- Secondary cyst formation from traumatic or surgical epithelial implantation

- Solid iris tumors

- Ciliary body tumors

Treatment

- Surgical excision with sector iridectomy may be preferred treatment because it may lessen risk of cyst leakage causing iritis and increased IOP and better the chance of removing entire tumor, lessening the chance of recurrence.

Prognosis

- Guarded

REFERENCES

Casey M, Cohen KL, Wallace DK. Recurrence of iris stromal cyst following aspiration and resection. *J AAPOS.* 2002;6(4):255–256.

Shields JA. Primary cysts of the iris. *Trans Am Ophthalmol Soc.* 1981;79: 771–809.

Shields JA, Shields CL, Lois N, et al. Iris cysts in children: classification, incidence and management: the 1998 Torrence A Makley Jr. lecture. *Br J Ophthalmol.* 1999;83(3):334–338.

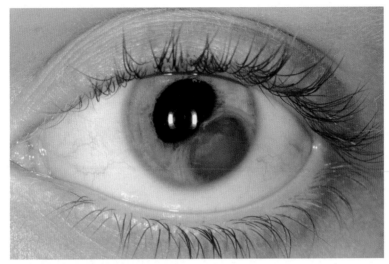

FIGURE 4-8. Whitish clear-appearing cyst in iris stroma. (Courtesy of Jerry Shields, MD.)

JUVENILE XANTHOGRANULOMA

Etiology

- Disorder of unknown etiology characterized by abnormal proliferation of non-Langerhans' histiocytes with Touton giant cells occurring predominantly in infancy and early childhood

- Most often occurs unilaterally

- Common in children with neurofibromatosis type 1 (NF1)

- Optic nerve, retina, and choroid can also be infiltrated

Symptoms

- May cause spontaneous hyphema with decreased vision and increased IOP, corneal enlargement, and perilimbal flush and photophobia

- Children with skin lesions of JXG are routinely screened for eye involvement.

Signs

- Can present as vascular, discrete reddish or yellow lesions or diffusely causing heterochromia irides (Fig. 4-9)

- Spontaneous or recurrent unilateral hyphema

- Skin lesions appear as an acquired tan or orange papule or nodule. Skin lesions are self-limited.

Differential Diagnosis

- Leukemic infiltrates

- Lisch nodules

- Brushfield spots

- Iris mamillations

Treatment

- Biopsy of skin lesion to confirm diagnosis in patients with concomitant skin lesions

- Anterior chamber paracentesis can be performed in patients without skin lesions.

- Avoid iris biopsy because of the high risk of hemorrhage.

- Topical or subconjunctival steroids can be used as the first line of treatment.

- Radiotherapy (with dose not exceeding 500 cGy) can be used if the initial treatment is unsuccessful and the risk-to-benefit ratio is acceptable.

Prognosis

- Good with timely and appropriate diagnosis and treatment

REFERENCES

DeBarge LR, Chan CC, Greenberg SC, et al. Chorioretinal, iris, and ciliary body infiltration by juvenile xanthogranuloma masquerading as uveitis. *Surv Ophthalmol.* 1994;39(1):65–71.

Shields CL, Shields JA, Buchanon HW. Solitary orbital involvement with juvenile xanthogranuloma. *Arch Ophthalmol.* 1990;108(11):1587–1589.

Zamir E, Wang RC, Krishnakumar S, et al. Juvenile xanthogranuloma masquerading as pediatric chronic uveitis: a clinicopathologic study. *Surv Ophthalmol.* 2001;46(2):164–171.

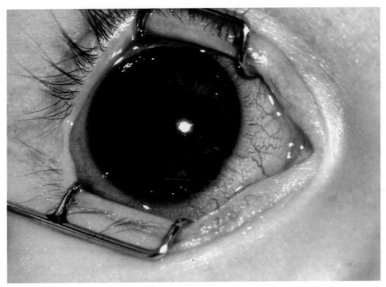

FIGURE 4-9. Reddish-yellow lesions on iris with signs of past intraocular inflammation. (Courtesy of Alex V. Levin, MD, MHSc, Wills Eye Institute, Philadelphia.)

LISCH NODULES

Etiology

- Discrete dome-shaped nodules, which are melanocytic hamartomas occurring in patients with NF1

- Occurs in children affected with NF1 at an incidence approximately equal to 10 times the child's age in years up to age 9 years

- Rare in NF2

Symptoms

- Nodules do not affect vision directly.

Signs

- Bilaterally occurring, discrete dome-shaped nodules appearing anywhere on the anterior iris surface (including the angle when gonioscopic observation may be necessary to see them) (Fig. 4-10)

- Most are round, mildly pigmented (tan), and may be distributed more on the inferior iris surface than the superior iris surface

- NF1 sometimes associated with pulsatile exophthalmos secondary to absence of the greater wing of the sphenoid bone and plexiform neuroma of the eyelid, giving an S-shaped deformity to the upper eyelid in early childhood

Differential Diagnosis

- Iris nevi
- Brushfield's spots
- JXG
- Iris mamillations

Treatment

- Observation of Lisch nodules in a child not carrying the diagnosis of NF should trigger a workup for the disease and evaluation of family members.

Prognosis

- Depends on the presence of absence of concomitant abnormalities associated with NF, such as optic nerve glioma

REFERENCES

Friedman JM. Neurofibromatosis 1. In: Pagon RA, Bird TC, Dolan CR, Stephens K, eds. *GeneReviews*. Seattle: University of Washington; 2009.

Jett K, Friedman JM. Clinical and genetic aspects of neurofibromatosis 1 [review]. *Genet Med.* 2010;12(1):1–11.

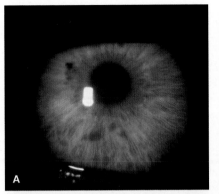
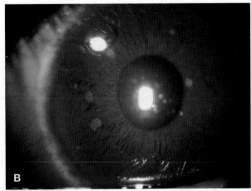
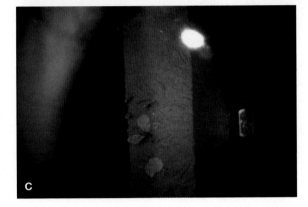

FIGURE 4-10. Discrete, mildly pigmented dome-shaped nodules on anterior iris surface of a white patient (**A**) and an African American patient (**B**). **C.** Slit-lamp photo of Lisch nodules on the anterior iris surface of an African American patient.

MELANOSIS OCULI (OCULAR MELANOCYTOSIS)

Etiology

- Congenital

- Increase in the number of melanocytes in the iris, sclera, uvea, and surrounding tissues. The melanocytes are located deep within the sclera, yielding a slate-gray pigmentation rather than the normal brownish pigmentation usually associated with melanin.

Symptoms

- Increased pigmentation of the iris; discoloration of the sclera

- Usually none unless associated with increased IOP or malignant melanoma

Signs

- A congenital, flat, slate-gray discoloration of the sclera, iris, and uveal tract (Fig. 4-11). The conjunctiva is not involved.

- Most often unilateral but can occur bilaterally

- Eyelid skin may be involved as well. Some patients, especially those of Asian ancestry, may have associated increased pigmentation of the eyelid and adjacent skin (oculodermal melanocytosis, nevus of Ota), which can appear brown, bluish, or black without another skin abnormality (Fig. 4-12).

Differential Diagnosis

- Bilateral patches of slate-gray scleral pigmentation common in Asian and African American children (which have no clinical significance)

- Congenital nevocellular nevus of the eyelids

- Conjunctival nevi

- Melanosis of the sclera and skin sometimes associated with Sturge-Weber syndrome and Klippel-Trenaunay-Weber syndrome

Treatment

- Increased risk of glaucoma and malignant melanoma occurs with increased intraocular pigmentation.

- Routine screening for glaucoma and yearly dilated fundus examination to rule out uveal melanoma

Prognosis

- Depends on the presence or absence of glaucoma and malignant melanoma

REFERENCES

Ellis FD. Selected pigmented fundus lesions of children. *J AAPOS*. 2005;9(4):306–314.

Honavar SG, Shields CL, Singh AD, et al. Two discrete choroidal melanomas in an eye with ocular melanocytosis [review]. *Surv Ophthalmol*. 2002;47(1):36–341.

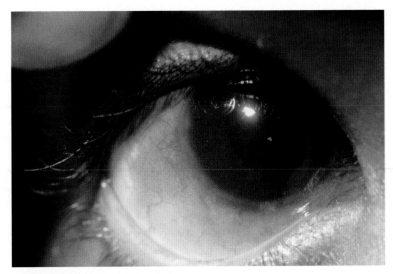

FIGURE 4-11. Flat, slate-gray discoloration of sclera.

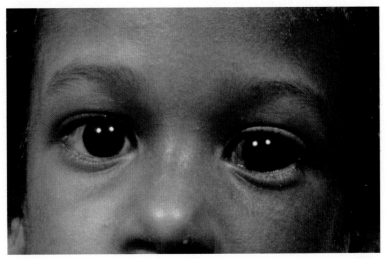

FIGURE 4-12. Oculodermal melanocytosis. Note the increased pigmentation of the sclera, eyelids, and adjacent skin on the left side.

PERSISTENT PUPILLARY MEMBRANE

Etiology

- Common developmental abnormality of the iris

- Results from incomplete involution of anterior tunic vasculosa lentis (which normally begins to involute at the beginning of the third trimester)

Symptoms

- Visually insignificant in almost all but most severely involved eyes

Signs

- Membranes attach to iris collarette, may be free floating or span the pupil and attach on the opposite side to the iris or to the anterior lens surface (which may be extensive) (Fig. 4-13)

- Can be associated with cataract (usually centrally located), microcornea, megalocornea, microphthalmos, and coloboma

Differential Diagnosis

- Fibrinous anterior uveitis

- Ectopia lentis et pupillae

Treatment

- In the rare cases when vision is effected by persistent papillary membranes, medical therapy (papillary dilation and amblyopia therapy) is usually adequate.

- Surgical intervention (including iridectomy, removal of membrane, and laser therapy) have been attempted in the past with mixed success.

Prognosis

- Usually very good without treatment

REFERENCES

Kothari M, Mody K. Excision of persistent pupillary membrane using a suction cutter. *J Pediatr Ophthalmol Strabismus.* 2009;46(3):187.

Kurt E. A patient with bilateral persistent pupillary membrane: a conservative approach. *J Pediatr Ophthalmol Strabismus.* 2009;46(5):300–302.

Meyer-Rüsenberg B, Thill M, Vujancevic S, et al. Conservative management of bilateral persistent pupillary membranes with 18 years of follow-up. *Graefes Arch Clin Exp Ophthalmol.* 2010;248(7):1053–1054.

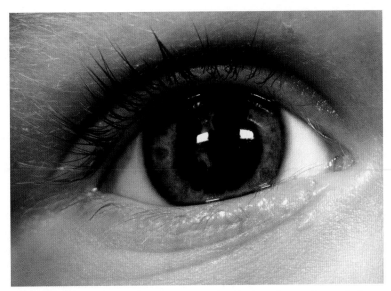

FIGURE 4-13. Persistent pupillary membrane spanning the pupil and attaching to the anterior lens surface. (Courtesy of Alex V. Levin, MD, MHSc, Wills Eye Institute, Philadelphia.)

POSTERIOR SYNECHIAE

Etiology

• Congenital adhesions from the iris margin to the lens capsule. Congenital adhesions may occur in association with cataract, intrauterine inflammation, and aniridia May also represent isolated remnants of the tunica vasculosa lentis (which are benign).

• Acquired adhesions occur more frequently and are most often associated with iridocyclitis.

Symptoms

• Patients are typically asymptomatic unless associated iridocyclitis or active sarcoidosis is present.

Signs

• Misshaped pupil

• Adhesions between the iris margin and lens capsule (Fig. 4-14)

• Congenital synechia may be associated with small anterior polar cataract at the point where the iris inserts into the lens capsule.

• Pigment on anterior lens capsule surface in a circular pattern often present after intraocular inflammation synechia are broken.

Differential Diagnosis

• Persistent pupillary membrane

• Acquired synechia can also be associated with sarcoidosis, with Koeppe or Busacca nodules.

Treatment

• Congenital synechia with anterior polar cataract may be associated with hyperopia astigmatism and anisometropic amblyopia.

• Pharmacologic treatment with eye drops to dilate the pupil can often successfully break fresh acquired synechia.

• Surgical synechialysis sometimes required when posterior synechia are present for a significant amount of the circumference of the papillary aperture or risk of angle closure is present.

REFERENCES

Kadayifçilar S, Eldem B, Tumer B. Uveitis in childhood. *J Pediatr Ophthalmol Strabismus*. 2003;40(6):335–340.

Levy-Clarke GA, Nussenblatt RB, Smith JA. Management of chronic pediatric uveitis [review]. *Curr Opin Ophthalmol*. 2005;16(5):281–288.

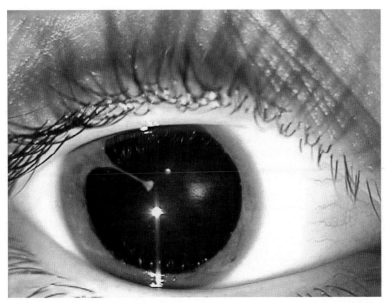

FIGURE 4-14. Adhesion between iris and anterior lens surface. (Courtesy of Jonathan Salvin, MD.)

AXENFELD-RIEGER ANOMALY

Etiology

- Part of a group of anterior segment defects (formerly known as mesodermal dysgenesis) with both genotypic and phenotypic overlap

- Iris and pupil abnormalities associated with anterior displacement of Schwalbe's line with iris bands extending to the cornea (Axenfeld's anomaly)

- Autosomal dominant inheritance most common

- Called Rieger's syndrome if associated with dental and skeletal abnormalities

- Mutations in *RIEG1/PITX2* gene (gene that regulates expansion of other genes during embryological development) on chromosome 4q25 has been identified.

- Mutations in FOXC1 (transcription factor gene) also associated

Symptoms

- Abnormally shaped iris or pupil

- Photophobia secondary to significant iridodysgenesis

Signs

- Prominent iris processes that insert to an anteriorly displaced Schwalbe's line (Fig. 4-15); may have a thinned iris stroma, bilateral iridodysgenesis with iris transillumination, peripheral anterior synechia, an eccentric and displaced pupil

Differential Diagnosis

- Posterior embryotoxon

- Peters' anomaly

- Ectopic pupil

Treatment

- 50% risk of glaucoma development; timely and appropriate monitoring for the development of glaucoma, including gonioscopy

- No treatment for underlying abnormalities

- Appropriate sunwear for photophobia symptoms

- Colored contact lens for glare and cosmesis concerns

- Genetic evaluation if systemic involvement is suspected

Prognosis

- Depends on involvement of the anterior segment and the presence of glaucoma

REFERENCES

Cella W, de Vasconcellos JP, de Melo MB, et al. Structural assessment of PITX2, FOXC1, CYP1B1, and GJA1 genes in patients with Axenfeld-Rieger syndrome with developmental glaucoma. *Invest Ophthalmol Vis Sci.* 2006;47(5):1803–1809.

Singh DV, Sharma YR, Azad RV, et al. Familial ectopia lentis with Axenfeld-Rieger anomaly. *J Pediatr Ophthalmol Strabismus.* 2007;44(1):59–61.

Yi K, Walden PG, Chen TC. What's your diagnosis? Axenfeld-Rieger anomaly without glaucoma. *J Pediatr Ophthalmol Strabismus.* 2007;44(6):333, 355.

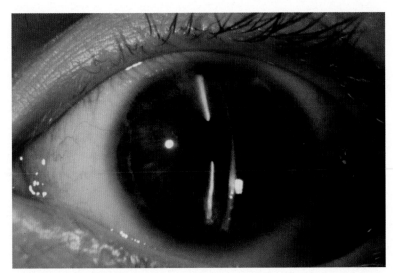

FIGURE 4-15. Iris processes inserting to an anteriorly displaced Schwalbe's line. (Courtesy of Alex V. Levin, MD, MHSc, Wills Eye Institute, Philadelphia.)

CHAPTER 5

Lens Anomalies

CONGENITAL AND DEVELOPMENTAL CATARACTS

Jonathan H. Salvin and Hillary Gordon ■

Cataracts are an opacification of the lens of the eye, typically associated with age. Congenital cataracts may present at or soon after birth, whereas developmental cataracts present during childhood. They may be unilateral or bilateral and may result in decreased visual acuity or blindness from the opacification and subsequent amblyopia (**Fig. 5-1**).

Etiology

- The prevalence is 1 to 15 per 10,000 children.
- Idiopathic (60% bilateral cases, 80% unilateral cases)
- Familial (30% cases)
- Genetic and metabolic diseases associated with cataract
  - Galactosemia
  - Alport's syndrome
  - Fabry's disease
  - Myotonic dystrophy
  - Diabetes mellitus
  - Trisomy 21
  - Trisomy 18
  - Trisomy 13
- Systemic illnesses associated with cataract include:
  - Juvenile idiopathic arthritis
  - Systemic lupus erythematosus
  - Malignancies
- Ocular abnormalities associated with cataract include:
  - Aniridia
  - Persistent hyperplastic primary vitreous (PHPV)
  - Anterior segment dysgenesis
- Maternal infection associated with cataract include:
  - Rubella
  - Cytomegalovirus
  - Varicella
  - Herpes simplex virus
  - Toxoplasmosis
  - Syphilis

Signs and Symptoms

- Variable lens opacity from small white spots in pupils to complete leukocoria
- Decreased visual acuity
- Asymmetric, diminished, or absent red reflex
- Nystagmus
- Photophobia
- Failure to meet developmental milestones
- Poor visual development in infants

Diagnostic Evaluation

- Detailed history with specific attention to family history, trauma, systemic steroid use, radiation exposure, maternal infection, systemic illness in child, and visual developmental milestones or visual changes
- Physical examination includes complete ophthalmologic examination with pupillary dilation, retinoscopy, slit-lamp examination, and visual acuity testing and indirect ophthalmoscopy
- B-scan ultrasonography
- Infants may require general anesthesia for full examination.
- Full physical examination with attention paid to growth and developmental milestones and appropriate referral for genetic, infectious, and metabolic testing

Treatment

- Cataract >3 mm, dense nuclear cataract, and cataract preventing full refraction or associated with nystagmus or strabismus are indications for surgery with or without intraocular lens replacement.

- In children younger than 7 years of age, treatment should be initiated within weeks after diagnosis to avoid the development of amblyopia.
- Partial cataracts may require surgery or may be managed medically depending on the extent of the cataract and the surgical risks. If visual acuity can accurately be measured to better than 20/50, pupillary dilation can be attempted for management. If the visual acuity cannot be accurately measured or is measure to be 20/50 or worse, surgery should be considered.
- Postoperative aphakic refractive correction (glasses or contact lenses) immediately after surgery
- Amblyopia treatment after cataract extraction
- Appropriate referral of patient for evaluation and treatment of any underlying disease

Prognosis

- Depends on the age at development diagnosis, treatment of the cataract, the type of cataract, the laterality, and surgical complications
- In young children, postoperative prognosis depends on adherence to amblyopia treatment.

REFERENCES

Amaya L, Taylor D, Russell-Eggitt I, et al. The morphology and natural history of childhood cataracts. *Surv Ophthalmol.* 2003;48:125–144.

Lim Z, Rubab S, Chan YH, et al. Pediatric cataract: the Toronto experience-etiology. *Am J Ophthalmol.* 2010; 149(6):887–892.

Lin AA, Buckley EG. Update on pediatric cataract surgery and intraocular lens implantation. *Curr Opin Ophthalmol.* 2010;21(1):55–59.

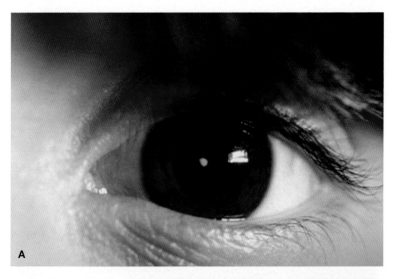

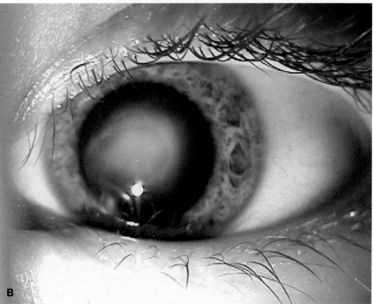

FIGURE 5-1. **A.** Anterior polar cataract: central anterior lens opacity generally less than 1 mm in diameter. These are rarely visually significant. **B.** Congenital nuclear cataract: large central nuclear opacity. This cataract is visually significant and requires surgical removal.

(*continued*)

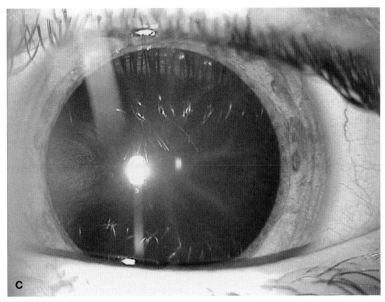

FIGURE 5-1. (*Continued*) **C.** Stellate congenital cataract: stellate, spokelike cortical lens opacity. Initially, this may not be visually significant, but it may progress to a total opacity.

ECTOPIA LENTIS

Hillary Gordon and Jonathan H. Salvin ▓

- Ectopia lentis is a displacement of the lens of the eye (**Fig. 5-2**). Subluxation is defined as partial dislocation with the lens remaining attached to ciliary body by the lens zonules. Luxation is the complete detachment of the lens from the ciliary body.

Etiology

- Trauma
- Congenital
- Ocular conditions
  - Simple ectopia lentis
  - Ectopia lentis et pupillae
  - Spherophakia
  - Aniridia
  - Iris coloboma
  - Congenital glaucoma
  - Retinitis pigmentosa
  - Rieger's syndrome
- Systemic diseases associated with ectopia lentis:
  - Marfan's syndrome
  - Homocystinuria
  - Weil-Marchesani syndrome
  - Ehlers-Danlos syndrome
  - Sulfite oxidase deficiency
  - Hyperlysinemia
  - Congenital syphilis
  - Crouzon's syndrome
  - Apert's disease

Symptoms

- Mild to severely decreased visual acuity due to progressive or acute changes in refractive error

- Pain associated with pupillary block glaucoma

Signs

- Partial lens displacement posteriorly or anteriorly
- Complete lens displacement into anterior chamber or posterior pole
- Pupillary block glaucoma
- Induced irregular refractive errors (irregular astigmatism, high myopia, or aphakia)
- Amblyopia
- Iridodonesis

Diagnostic Evaluation

- Detailed history to determine the etiology with special attention paid to recent head, orbit, or eye trauma
- Full ocular exam including visual acuity, slit-lamp examination, and dilated fundoscopic examination
- Appropriate genetic, metabolic, and/or infectious studies if trauma ruled out

Treatment

- Refractive correction with corrective lenses
- Amblyopia management
- Lensectomy with postoperative aphakic glasses or contact lenses
- Lensectomy with intraocular lens implantation (IOL) if possible
- Treatment of secondary ocular conditions (i.e., pupillary block glaucoma)
- Refer to appropriate specialist for evaluation and treatment of underlying medical condition.

Prognosis

- 90% of patients have a visual acuity of 20/40 or better after surgery with appropriate refractive correction.

REFERENCES

Colley A, Lloyd IC, Ridgway A, et al. Ectopia lentis et pupillae; the genetic aspects and differential diagnosis. *J Med Genet.* 1991;28(11):791–794.

Neely DE, Plager DA. Management of ectopia lentis in children. *Ophthalmol Clin North Am.* 2001; 14(3):493–499.

Young TL. Ophthalmic genetics/inherited eye disease. *Curr Opin Ophthalmol.* 2003;14(5):296–303.

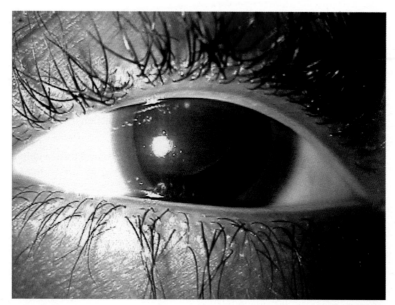

FIGURE 5-2. Ectopia lentis: lens dislocation in the superonasal direction more typically seen in Marfan's syndrome.

ANTERIOR LENTICONUS

Jonathan H. Salvin ■

Anterior lenticonus is an anterior bowing of the anterior capsule of the lens, often with associated lens opacification. (Fig. 5-3)

Etiology

- May be associated with anterior subcapsular or anterior polar cataracts

- Alport's syndrome, an inherited disorder (X-linked in 85%) with hemorrhagic nephritis and sensorineural hearing loss

- Trauma

Symptoms

- If small (<2–3 mm), no symptoms

- If larger, then blurred vision or induced amblyopia

Signs

- Typically bilateral

- Central, conical anterior protrusion of the anterior lens capsule seen on slit-lamp examination (Fig. 5-3)

- Central "oil-drop" appearance on red reflex examination

- Induced myopic or astigmatic refractive errors

Diagnosis

- Detailed history, including family history for Alport's syndrome

- Complete eye examination, including visual acuity, slit-lamp examination, dilated fundoscopic examination, retinoscopy, and refraction

- Referral for appropriate nephrology and hearing evaluation

Treatment

- Refractive correction

- Amblyopia management

- Pharmacologic pupillary dilation for small capsular irregularity or opacity

- Cataract extraction if visually significant opacity

- Clear lensectomy if unable to improve vision with refractive correction or pupillary dilation alone

- Treatment of underlying systemic nephrology disease

- Hearing loss management

Prognosis

- Good vision is achievable with close observation and cataract extraction when indicated.

REFERENCES

Flinter F. Alport's syndrome. *J Med Genet.* 1997;34: 326–330.

Trivedi R, Wilson ME. Anterior lenticonus in Alport syndrome. In: Wilson ME, Trivedi R, Pandey S, eds. *Pediatric Cataract Surgery.* Philadelphia: Lippincott Williams & Wilkins; 2005:194–198.

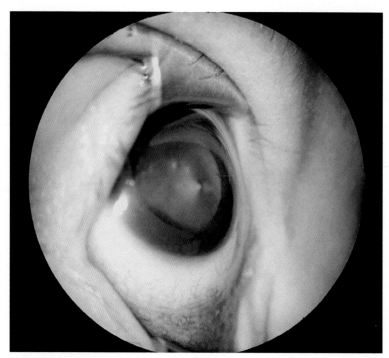

FIGURE 5-3. Anterior lenticonus.

POSTERIOR LENTICONUS

Jonathan H. Salvin ■

Posterior lenticonus is a thinning of the posterior capsule with an associated posterior bowing of the central lens capsule (**Fig. 5-4**). Typically, the posterior lens opacifications are progressive and become full posterior subsupcasular cataracts. Often at the time of cataract surgery, there is an associated hole in the posterior capsule that may lead to vitreous prolapse during surgery.

Etiology

● Congenital

Symptoms

● Often no symptoms early

● Decreased vision with progression

Signs

● Posterior lens changes seen on slit-lamp examination or red reflex testing

● Amblyopia

● Irregular lenticular astigmatism

Diagnosis

● Detailed history

● Complete eye examination, including visual acuity, slit-lamp examination, dilated fundoscopic examination, retinoscopy, and refraction

Treatment

● Observation

● Amblyopia management

● Refractive correction

● Lensectomy with special care taken in managing the posterior capsule during surgery; many of these patients have a posterior capsular defect at the time of surgery

Prognosis

● Generally good even after cataract surgery

REFERENCES

Amaya L, Taylor D, Russell-Eggitt I, et al. The morphology and natural history of childhood cataracts. *Surv Ophthalmol*. 2003;48:125–144.

Khali M, Saheb N. Posterior lenticonus. *Ophthalmology*. 1984;91:1429–1430.

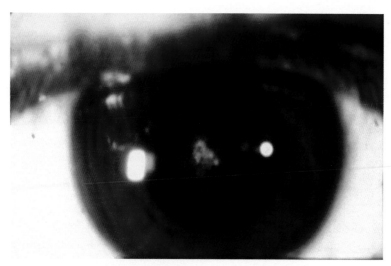

FIGURE 5-4. Posterior lenticonus: posterior lens opacification. Early, this may not be visually significant, but may progress to complete posterior subcapsular opacity.

SPHEROPHAKIA

Jonathan H. Salvin ▮

Spherophakia is when the lens has a spherical shape with increased lens thickness and increased curvature and resultant lenticular myopia. Microspherophakia is when the lens is spherical and smaller and is associated with the increased risk of dislocation (ectopia lentis) (Fig. 5-5).

Etiology

- Idiopathic or congenital
- Weill-Marchesani syndrome
- Marfan's syndrome

Symptoms

- Mild to severely decreased visual acuity caused by progressive or acute changes in refractive error
- Pain associated with pupillary block glaucoma

Signs

- High lenticular myopia
- Irregular astigmatism
- Amblyopia
- Pupillary block glaucoma
- Anterior or posterior lens dislocation

Diagnosis

- Detailed history to determine the etiology with special attention paid to recent head, orbit, or eye trauma
- Full ocular examination, including visual acuity, slit-lamp examination, and dilated fundoscopic examination
- Appropriate genetic, metabolic, and infectious studies if trauma ruled out

Treatment

- Refractive correction
- Amblyopia management
- Lensectomy with postoperative aphakic glasses or contact lenses
- Lensectomy with IOL if possible
- Treatment of secondary ocular conditions (i.e., pupillary block glaucoma)
- Refer to appropriate specialist for evaluation and treatment of underlying medical condition

REFERENCES

Jensen AD, Cross HE, Paton D. Ocular complications in the Weill-Marchesani syndrome. *Am J Ophthalmol.* 1974;77:261–269.

Ritch R, Chang BM, Liebmann JM. Angle closure in younger patients. *Ophthalmology.* 2003;110: 1880–1889.

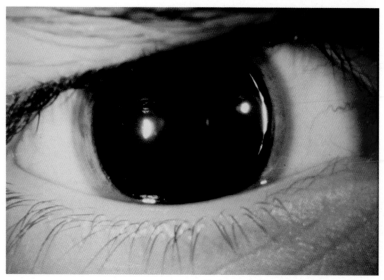

FIGURE 5-5. Patient with microspherophakia. The small and spherical lens edge is visible nasally. (Courtesy of Alex Levin, MD.)

Retinal Anomalies

BEST'S DISEASE

Barry N. Wasserman ■

Etiology

● An autosomal dominant disorder also called *vitelliform macular dystrophy*, Best's disease leads to retinal pigment epithelium (RPE) degeneration and secondary loss of photoreceptors in the macula.

● Mutations lead to abnormal bestrophin, a Ca^{2+} sensitive Cl^- channel protein. Lipofuscin accumulates in the RPE cells, yielding a characteristic "egg yolk" appearance (hence the name vitelliform) in the fovea and macula. Multifocal lesions may also occur.

Symptoms

● Early in the disease process, patients may be asymptomatic, but later metamorphopsia and deceased visual acuity occur.

● Symptoms are variable and may be asymmetric, with significant vision loss in adulthood.

Signs

● Stages are described based on phenotypic appearance in the macula, which may be asymmetric between the eyes. Earliest stage disease may only reveal subtle RPE mottling or may be normal. Later yellow orange material collects in the macula as a 0.5- to 5.0-mm diameter lesion yielding the classic "egg yolk" appearance. Clear fluid slowly builds around the lesion in the subretinal space, with resultant cystic appearance with fluid level (Fig. 6-1A). As this fluid dissipates, the lesion again changes to a more "scrambled egg"(vitelliruptive) stage, associated with pigment clumping (Fig. 6-1B). Later stages include atrophic changes with fibrosis, macular degeneration, and significant vision loss sometimes followed by choroidal neovascularization.

Differential Diagnosis

● Stargardt's disease
● Sorsby's macular dystrophy
● Pattern dystrophy
● North Carolina macular dystrophy
● Solar retinopathy

- Coalescence of basal laminar drusen
- Central serous retinopathy with fibrinous exudate
- Pigment epithelial detachment of age-related macular degeneration
- Adult foveomacular dystrophy
- Age-related macular degeneration

Diagnostic Evaluation

- Diagnosis is based on clinical findings along with electrophysiologic studies revealing normal electroretinogram and abnormal electro-oculogram. In addition, there is high autofluorescence.
- Optical coherence tomography (OCT) detects subretinal deposits and fluid.
- Genetic studies may reveal mutation in the bestrophin gene.

Treatment

- There is no treatment for early disease, but late choroidal neovascularization has been treated with intravitreal injection of bevacizumab.

- Genetic counseling and examination of family members are recommended, as are low vision and occupational consultations.

Prognosis

- Some patients maintain good vision (20/40) throughout life.
- In others, good vision (20/20–20/50) usually persists through the early stages but decreases to 20/200 in the fifth and sixth decades of life as the atrophic and cicatricial stages progress.

REFERENCES

Goodwin P. Hereditary retinal disease. *Curr Opin Ophthalmol.* 2008;19:255–262.

Leu J, Schrage NF, Degenring RF. Choroidal neovascularisation secondary to Best's disease in a 13-year-old boy treated by intravitreal bevacizumab. *Graefes Arch Clin Exp Ophthalmol.* 2007;245(11):1723–1725.

Spaide RF, Noble K, Morgan A, et al. Vitelliform macular dystrophy. *Ophthalmology.* 2006;113:1392–1400.

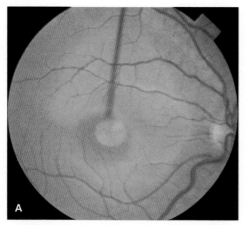 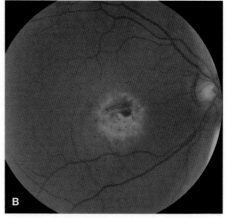

FIGURE 6-1. A. Best's disease with early macular "egg yolk" appearance. **B.** Best's disease with later "scrambled egg" appearance.

CHOROIDEREMIA

Barry N. Wasserman ■

Etiology

- An X-linked recessive disease, choroideremia is a progressive retinal degeneration. Males show loss of choriocapillaris and RPE. Female carriers can show mild signs of the disease, with patchy retinal abnormalities and corresponding visual field defects caused by lyonization, but are generally asymptomatic.

- Mutation in the *CHM* gene affects production of the Rab escort protein 1 (REP-1). Degeneration begins in the midperiphery and progresses both centrally toward the macula and toward the periphery.

Symptoms

- Patients present in the first two decades of life with early loss of night vision and peripheral vision.

- Central vision may be maintained until around the fifth decade of life but is eventually lost.

Signs

- Retinal examination reveals loss of the RPE and choriocapillaris with exposure of the larger choroidal vessels (**Fig. 6-2**). Remaining RPE may have a salt and pepper appearance.

- Later in the disease, large areas of exposed sclera may be seen on funduscopy. Posterior subcapsular cataracts may be associated.

Differential Diagnosis

- Advanced retinitis pigmentosa
- Gyrate atrophy
- Pathologic myopia
- Chorioretinitis (e.g., acute retinal necrosis, after cytomegalovirus [CMV] retinitis)

Diagnostic Evaluation

- X-linked inheritance with typical fundus appearance in affected males.

- Visual field testing demonstrates constriction.

- Fluorescein angiography reveals large choroidal vessels caused by loss of overlying RPE and choriocapillaris.

- Electroretinography may be consistent with a rod-cone dystrophy early in the disease but eventually becomes extinguished.

- Genetic analysis to assess mutation in the *CHM* gene may be performed, and analysis of peripheral blood is available to demonstrate absence of the Rab escort protein 1. Female carriers may demonstrate patches of irregular pigmentation in the RPE.

Treatment

- Genetic counseling for family members should be suggested.

- Low vision evaluation and treatment may be helpful.

- Gene therapy has shown some success in animal models.

Prognosis

- Patients progressively lose night and peripheral vision.

- Central vision is often maintained into adulthood but is ultimately lost.

REFERENCES

Lee TK, McTaggart KE, Sieving PA, et al. Clinical diagnoses that overlap with choroideremia. *Can J Ophthalmol.* 2003;38(5):364–372.

MacDonald IM, Russell L, Chan CC. Choroideremia: new findings from ocular pathology and review of recent literature. *Surv Ophthalmol.* 2009;54(3):401–407.

MacDonald IM, Smaoui N, Seabra MC. Choroideremia. In: Pagon RA, Bird TC, Dolan CR, et al, eds. *GeneReviews.* Seattle: University of Washington; 2010.

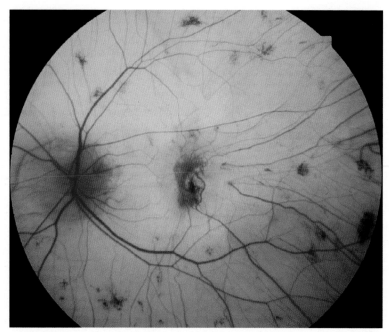

FIGURE 6-2. Choroideremia at advanced stage, with complete loss of retinal pigment epithelium and choriocapillaris.

GYRATE ATROPHY

Barry N. Wasserman ■

Etiology

- Gyrate atrophy is an autosomal recessive disease caused by a deficiency of the mitochondrial enzyme, ornithine aminotransferase.

- Elevated ornithine levels are toxic to the RPE, causing gradual loss of peripheral vision and night vision.

- Mutations of the ornithine aminotransferase gene (10q26) have been identified.

Symptoms

- Nyctalopia and loss of visual field may begin in the first two decades of life but may not be manifest until the fifth decade. The disease affects both eyes symmetrically.

- Central vision is spared usually until the fourth or fifth decade but then declines.

- Symptoms and signs may vary widely in patients in all age groups.

Signs

- Fundus examination early in the disease shows scalloped areas of geographic atrophic RPE and choriocapillaris (**Fig. 6-3**).

- The macula is relatively spared until late in the disease, although epiretinal membranes and cystoid macular edema can occur.

- Patients may have cataracts and myopia.

Differential Diagnosis

- Choroideremia
- Retinitis pigmentosa
- Choroidal atrophy
- Chorioretinitis (e.g., acute retinal necrosis, following CMV retinitis)

Diagnostic Evaluation

- Ocular examination may reveal mildly decreased visual acuity, and refractive error is commonly myopic.

- Cataracts may be seen on slit-lamp evaluation.

- Funduscopy shows mid peripheral and peripheral scalloped geographic areas of RPE and choriocapillaris. Areas of intact RPE may have increased pigmentation.

- The macula is usually spared early in the disease, but cystoid macular edema may be demonstrated with OCT.

- Optic atrophy and attenuated retinal vessels are seen later in the disease.

- Visual fields are markedly constricted, and electroretinography reveals absent photopic and scotopic responses.

- Plasma ornithine levels are markedly elevated.

Treatment

- Genetic counseling is suggested.

- A diet restricting arginine will lower the plasma ornithine and may slow the loss of visual function.

- Low vision services should be recommended.

Prognosis

- Although dietary arginine restriction delays the loss of function, the macula is eventually effected in most patients.

REFERENCES

Kaiser-Kupfer MI, Caruso RC, Valle D, et al. Use of an arginine-restricted diet to slow progression of visual loss in patients with gyrate atrophy. *Arch Ophthalmol.* 2004;122:982–984.

Peltola KE, Nanto-Salonen K, Heinonen OJ, et al. Ophthalmologic heterogeneity in subjects with gyrate atrophy of choroid and retina harboring the L402P mutation of ornithine aminotransferase. *Ophthalmology.* 2001;108:721–729.

Tamara TL, Andrade RE, Muccioli C, et al. Cystoid macular edema in gyrate atrophy of the choroid and retina: a fluorescein angiography and optical coherence tomography evaluation. *Am J Ophthalmol.* 2005;140: 147–149.

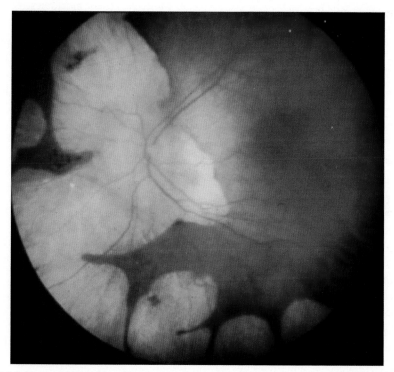

FIGURE 6-3. Gyrate atrophy with scalloped geographic atrophy of the retinal pigment epithelium and choriocapillaris. The macula is spared early in the disease.

LEBER CONGENITAL AMAUROSIS

Barry N. Wasserman

Etiology

- Leber congenital amaurosis is a severe congenital retinal dystrophy affecting both cones and rods. Vision is often less than 20/200.

- Mutations in more than 14 genes have been identified. The disease is almost autosomal recessive and rarely autosomal dominant.

Symptoms and Signs

- Patients present with nystagmus at 2 to 3 months old. Children show poor visual behavior, and some show self-stimulatory eye poking (oculodigital reflex).

- Pupils may be sluggish or paradoxical.

- Ophthalmoscopic findings are highly variable and may include a normal fundus appearance.

- Highly abnormal findings may also include chorioretinal atrophy, macular "coloboma" (Fig. 6-4A), retinal pigment epithelial irregularities, leopard spotting, nummular pigmentary abnormalities (Fig. 6-4B), and subretinal flecks.

- Retinal vessel attenuation and optic disc pallor are frequently present.

- Cataract, keratoconus, and strabismus may be associated findings.

Differential Diagnosis

- Achromatopsia
- Cone dystrophy
- Goldman-Favre disease
- Refsum phytanic acid storage disease
- Bassen-Kornzweig (abetalipoproteinemia) syndrome
- Juvenile retinal dystrophy
- Toxoplasmosis (when macular "coloboma" present)

Diagnostic Evaluation

- Family history may reveal consanguinity or distantly related affected individuals.

- Examination, including retinal evaluation, combined with extinguished electroretinography findings is diagnostic.

- Molecular genetic mutation screens are now available.

- Systemic and blood testing are important to rule out treatable causes, such as Refsum phytanic acid storage disease.

- Because there may be associated abnormalities of the kidneys, the liver, or hearing, appropriate testing is recommended.

Treatment

- Low vision evaluation and treatment can aid in function in some patients.

- Gene transfer via subretinal administration of adeno-associated viral (AAV) vectors encoding has demonstrated safety and in some cases efficacy for patients with mutations in the gene *RPE65*.

Prognosis

- Vision for most patients is poor.

- Future advances in gene therapy are promising.

REFERENCES

Goodwin P. Hereditary retinal disease. *Curr Opin Ophthalmol.* 2008;19:255–262.

Simonelli F, Maguire AM, Testa F, et al. Gene therapy for Leber's congenital amaurosis is safe and effective through 1.5 years after vector administration. *Mol Ther.* 2010;18(3):643–650.

Traboulsi EI. The Marshall M. Parks memorial lecture: making sense of early-onset childhood retinal dystrophies—the clinical phenotype of Leber congenital amaurosis. *Br J Ophthalmol.* 2010;94(10):1281–1287.

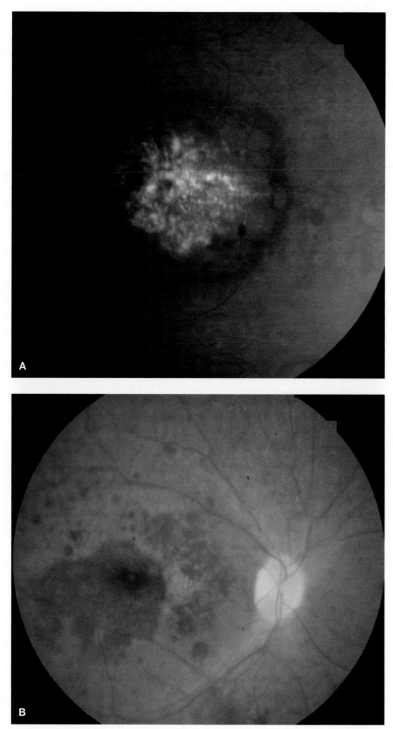

FIGURE 6-4. Leber congenital amaurosis with macular "coloboma" (**A**) and nummular pigmentary abnormalities (**B**).

ASTROCYTIC HAMARTOMA

Anuradha Ganesh ▪

● Retinal astrocytic hamartoma is a glial tumor arising from the retinal nerve fiber layer. It is most frequently associated with tuberous sclerosis (Bourneville's disease) but may very rarely be seen in neurofibromatosis or as an isolated ocular finding in otherwise normal individuals.

● Astrocytic hamartomas are believed to be congenital in most cases but may not be recognized until later in childhood. Patients with these lesions are usually asymptomatic.

Epidemiology and Etiology

● Most astrocytic hamartomas occur congenitally in association with tuberous sclerosis, a phakomatosis characterized by the triad of seizures, mental retardation, and skin lesions (Table 6-1).

● Tuberous sclerosis has an estimated incidence of 1 in 15,000 to 100,000 and exhibits autosomal dominant inheritance. About 60% of cases are spontaneous mutations. Mutations in either the *TSC1* or *TSC2* gene on chromosomes 9q34 and 16p13, respectively, result in tuberous sclerosis.

TABLE 6-1. Typical Manifestations of Tuberous Sclerosis

Skin lesions (<95% incidence)
   Hypomelanotic macules
   Facial angiofibromas (adenoma sebaceum)
Brain
   Seizures (<90% incidence)
   Developmental delay (<60% incidence)
Additional manifestations
   Periungual fibromas
   Pleural cysts and spontaneous pneumothorax
   Renal angiomyolipoma
   Cardiac rhabdomyoma
   Hamartomas of the liver, thyroid, pancreas, or testis

Signs

● About 50% of patients with tuberous sclerosis develop astrocytic hamartomas, approximately 50% of whom have bilateral involvement.

● Retinal astrocytic hamartomas are usually small, ranging from 0.5 to 5.0 mm in diameter, and are principally of two types: small, flat, smooth tumors that appear as subtle, ill-defined, semitranslucent thickening of the nerve fiber layer (Fig. 6-5A). Over time, they may become more opaque and contain calcification. Larger, opaque, calcified, sessile, whitish-yellow nodular masses ("mulberry lesion") are found at the optic nerve (Fig. 6-5B). Visual field testing may reveal a scotoma in the area corresponding to the tumor.

● Occasionally, lesions may produce vitreous hemorrhage, vitreous seeding, subretinal hemorrhage, or retinal detachment. The presence of yellow, lipoproteinaceous exudation in the sensory retina and subretinal space is an uncommon feature.

● Less frequent ocular manifestations include patches of iris or RPE hypopigmentation and hamartomas of the iris and ciliary body.

● Patients with an astrocytic hamartoma of the retina or optic nerve should be evaluated for tuberous sclerosis, which is characterized by the triad of skin lesions, seizures, and mental retardation. Additional manifestations include hamartomas in various organ systems. Diagnostic criteria for tuberous sclerosis facilitate identifying definite, probable, and possible cases).

Differential Diagnosis

● Retinoblastoma

● Retinocytoma

● Myelinated nerve fibers

● Retinal or optic nerve granuloma

● Drusen of the optic nerve

● Papillitis or papilledema

● Optic nerve infiltration (e.g., tuberculosis, sarcoid, leukemia)

Diagnostic Evaluation

- OCT: The astrocytic hamartoma replaces normal retinal architecture and appears as an optically hyperreflective mass with retinal disorganization, moth-eaten spaces, and posterior shadowing.

- Fluorescein angiography: The tumor appears relatively hypofluorescent in the arterial phase. Superficial find blood vessels are seen during the venous phase. The tumor stains intensely and homogeneously in the late phases. This test is rarely indicated.

- B-scan ultrasonography: A larger, calcified lesion often appears as a discrete, oval, solid mass with a sharp anterior border.

- Biopsy: In rare cases, differentiation from retinoblastoma (young patient) or choroidal melanoma (older patient) requires fine-needle aspiration biopsy

- Imaging or ultrasonography: To detect astrocytomas in the brain and other parts of the body, including the chest and abdomen.

Treatment and Prognosis

- Most cases of retinal astrocytoma are asymptomatic and do not require treatment.

- Rarely, some tumors can exhibit aggressive behavior and cause hemorrhage; retinal detachment; or even more uncommonly, neovascular glaucoma.

- Serial follow-up is indicated.

- Retinal detachment can be treated with demarcating laser photocoagulation.

- Progressive lesions may require measures such as endoresection; brachytherapy; and at times, enucleation.

- Family members should be examined for manifestations of tuberous sclerosis. Genetic testing may be useful in confirming the diagnosis and identifying affected relatives, allowing monitoring for early detection of problems associated with tuberous sclerosis, thus leading to earlier treatment and better outcomes.

REFERENCES

Northrup H, Sing Au K. Tuberous sclerosis complex Bourneville disease. In: Pagon RA, Bird TC, Dolan CR, et al, eds. *GeneReviews*. Seattle: University of Washington; 2009.

Roach ES, Sparagana SP. Diagnosis of tuberous sclerosis complex. *J Child Neurol*. 2004;19:643–649.

Shields CL, Benevides R, Materin MA, et al. Optical coherence tomography of retinal astrocytic hamartoma in 15 cases. *Ophthalmology*. 2006;113:1553–1557.

Shields JA, Eagle RC Jr, Shields CL, et al. Aggressive retinal astrocytomas in 4 patients with tuberous sclerosis complex, *Arch Ophthalmol*. 2005;123:856–863.

Shields JA, Shields CL. *Atlas of Intraocular Tumors*. Philadelphia: Lippincott Williams & Wilkins; 1999: 269–286.

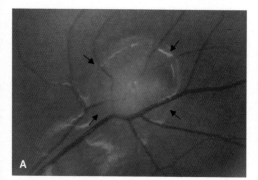 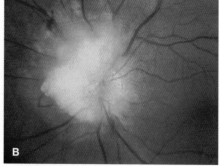

FIGURE 6-5. Astrocytic hamartoma. **A.** Small, ill-defined thickening of the nerve fiber layer. The *arrows* indicate the edge of the lesion. **B.** Large, opaque, calcified, sessile, whitish-yellow nodular mass ("mulberry lesion") at the optic nerve.

INCONTINENTIA PIGMENTI

Anuradha Ganesh and Alex V. Levin ■

• Incontinentia pigmenti, or Bloch-Sulzberger syndrome, is a rare X-linked dominant disorder of skin pigmentation that is accompanied by ocular, dental and central nervous system manifestations.

Epidemiology and Etiology

• The incidence of incontinentia pigmenti is 1 in 40,000 live births.

• In most cases, incontinentia pigmenti is caused by mutations in the *NEMO* (NF-κB essential modulator) gene at chromosome Xq28.

• As an X-linked dominant condition, it is usually lethal in males and thus usually only seen in female infants. An affected male with Klinefelter's syndrome (XXY) or genetic mosaicism may rarely survive.

• Incontinentia pigmenti refers to the histologic feature of "incontinence" of melanocytes in the basal layer of the epidermis of their pigment, which is then found in the superficial dermis.

History

• Characteristic skin lesions are usually present at birth.

• Ophthalmic findings are noted in infancy or sometimes later in life.

• A pedigree may reveal a history of male fetus miscarriages.

Signs

• The hallmark of ophthalmic involvement, present in more than 40% of patients, is peripheral retinal capillary nonperfusion (Fig. 6-6). This avascular retina may be demarcated by an intervening peripheral ring of neovascularization or otherwise abnormal retinal vessels, reminiscent of the clinical findings in retinopathy of prematurity (ROP). Retinal ischemia leads to the arteriovenous anastomoses and neovascularization. The disease may resolve spontaneously, but 10% of infants develop retinal folds, traction, and rhegmatogenous retinal detachment with consequent visual impairment. The ocular abnormalities are often asymmetric. Other eye findings are largely secondary and include strabismus in one third of infants, cataracts, and retinal pigmentary changes with mottled, diffuse hypopigmentation, and foveal hypoplasia.

• Skin findings include vesicular eruptions at birth that later evolve into desquamating erythematous lesions (Fig. 6-7A) followed by swirling hyperpigmentation (marble cake appearance; Fig. 6-7B) and then scarring.

• Dental abnormalities occur in more than 90% of affected individuals and include hypodontia; delayed eruption; and malformed, cone-shaped crowns. Associated central nervous system abnormalities include seizures, spastic paralysis, and mental retardation.

Differential Diagnosis

• ROP

• Familial exudative vitreoretinopathy (FEVR)

• Sickle cell disease (in older children)

• Other causes of infantile retinal nonattachment or detachment should also be considered.

Diagnostic Evaluation

• The diagnosis of incontinentia pigmenti is based on clinical criteria (Table 6-2). Tests that may help in confirming the diagnosis include skin biopsy (although there is a wide differential diagnosis for the findings described above), neuroimaging (cerebral atrophy, agenesis of corpus callosum), fluorescein angiography (avascular peripheral retina, anomalous vessels in vascular-avascular

TABLE 6-2. Diagnostic Criteria for Incontinentia Pigmenti*

Major Criteria

Four stages of skin lesions from infancy to adulthood:
A. Linear vesicles and bullae of stage 1
B. Dark brown colored verrucous papules and plaques of stage 2
C. Light brown colored swirling hyperpigmentation of stage 3
D. White atrophic patches of stage 4

Minor Criteria

A. Teeth: hypodontia, anodontia, or microdontia
B. Hair: alopecia, wiry hair
C. Nails: mild ridging or pitting
D. Retina: peripheral neovascularization

---

*The clinical diagnosis of incontinentia pigmenti can be made if at least one of the major criteria is present. The presence of minor criteria supports the clinical diagnosis; the complete absence of minor criteria should raise doubt regarding the diagnosis.
Adapted from Landy SJ, Donnai D. Incontinentia pigmenti (Bloch-Sulzberger syndrome). *J Med Genet.* 1993;30:53–59.

junction), and genetic testing (for mutations in the *NEMO* gene).

- Careful skin, dental, and ocular examination of the patient's mother may be useful as variable expression.

Treatment and Prognosis

- Patients with incontinentia pigmenti require careful retinal examination early in infancy to detect peripheral retinal non-perfusion. If present, frequent follow-up is indicated to enable early detection of change that might suggest development of retinal neovascularization, vascular leakage, and traction.

- No treatment is indicated unless such changes develop, in which case laser photocoagulation is performed in an effort to prevent progression to retinal traction and detachment.

- Genetic counseling is also highly recommended.

REFERENCES

Holmstrom G, Thoren K. Ocular manifestations of incontinentia pigmenti. *Acta Ophthalmol Scand.* 2000; 78:348–353.

International IP Consortium. Genomic rearrangement in NEMO impairs NF-kappaB activation and is a cause of incontinentia pigmenti. *Nature.* 2000;405:466–447.

Landy SJ, Donnai D. Incontinentia pigmenti (Bloch-Sulzberger syndrome). *J Med Genet.* 1993;30:53–59.

Scheuerle A, Ursini MV. Incontinentia pigmenti Bloch Sulzberger syndrome. In: Pagon RA, Bird TC, Dolan CR, et al, eds. *GeneReviews.* Seattle: University of Washington; 2005.

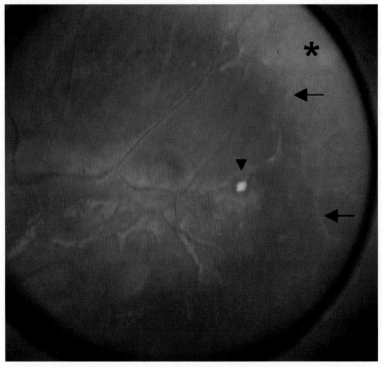

FIGURE 6-6. Fundus of a patient with incontinentia pigmenti showing peripheral retinal capillary nonperfusion (*asterisk*), arteriovenous anastomoses (*arrows*), and exudates (*arrowhead*).

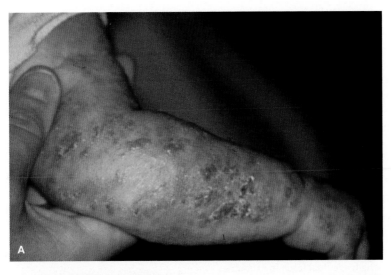

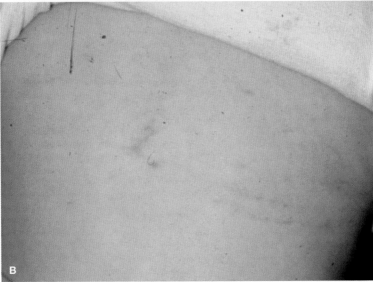

FIGURE 6-7. Skin findings in Coats' disease. Vesicular and desquamating erythematous lesions in an infant with incontinentia pigmenti (**A**) and swirling hyperpigmentation ("marble cake" appearance) (**B**).

COATS' DISEASE

Barry N. Wasserman and Carol L. Shields ■

Coats' disease is a nonhereditary condition characterized by unilateral retinal telangiectasia, exudation, and exudative retinal detachment that occurs most often in young patients.

Etiology

● Coats' disease is more common in males and generally occurs as a unilateral trait.

● The average age at onset is 2 to 8 years.

● Telangiectatic arterioles or venules lead to subretinal and intraretinal exudation of fluid and lipid, which eventual leads to exudative retinal detachment and vision loss.

● Some evidence indicates that Coats' disease is related to a somatic mutation in the Norrie's disease protein (NDP) gene or the frizzled 4 gene (*FZD4*).

Symptoms

● The symptoms include painless vision loss, particularly when the disease occurs at an older age.

● Younger patients often present with strabismus or xanthochroia.

● Rarely, patients manifest neovascular glaucoma and a red, painful eye.

● In an analysis of 150 cases of Coats' disease, the symptoms included decreased visual acuity (43%), strabismus (23%), xanthochroia (20%), pain (3%), heterochromia (1%), nystagmus (1%), and no symptoms (8%).

Signs

● The findings in Coats' disease include telangiectasia (100%), retinal exudation (99%), exudative retinal detachment (81%), retina hemorrhage (13%), retinal macrocyst (11%), vasoproliferative tumor (6%), and neovascularization of disc (2%), retina (1%), and iris (8%). Anterior chamber cholesterolosis occurs in 3%.

Differential Diagnosis

● Retinoblastoma
● ROP
● Retinal hemangioblastoma
● Retinal vasoproliferative tumor
● Sickle cell retinopathy
● FEVR
● Toxocariasis
● Leukemia
● Persistent fetal vasculature (PFV; persistent hyperplastic primary vitreous [PHPV])
● Radiation retinopathy
● Retinopathy of hypertensive crisis
● Cataract
● Coloboma

Diagnostic Evaluation

● The diagnosis is established by recognition of the clinical features on ophthalmoscopy. Retinal telangiectatic vessels with fusiform and nodular vascular dilation and adjacent nonperfusion are found, classically in the temporal quadrant. Related intraretinal and subretinal exudation is noted, and often retinal detachment is found (**Figs. 6-8 and 6-9**).

● Fluorescein angiography confirms these findings and additionally reveals vascular leakage and macular edema. The classification of Coats' disease, proposed by Shields et al, is:

■ Stage 1: retinal telangiectasia (T)
■ Stage 2: T + exudation (E)
■ Stage 3: T + E + subretinal fluid (F)
■ Stage 4: T + E + F + neovascular glaucoma (G)
■ Stage 5: T + E + F + G + phthisis bulbi

Treatment

● Laser photocoagulation or cryotherapy is used to obliterate leaking vessels.

● The role of intravitreal anti-VEGFs is being explored.

- Pars plana vitrectomy with drainage of subretinal fluid and exudation is used for advanced cases.

Prognosis

- The visual prognosis is often poor. In one analysis of 150 cases, poor visual acuity of 20/200 or worse was found in no patients with stage 1 disease, but 50% of stage 2, 70% of stage 3, and 100% of stage 4 and 5 patients showed poor vision.

- The goal of treatment is stabilization of the eye with resolution of retinal detachment and exudation and prevention of neovascular glaucoma and loss of the eye.

- There are no systemic implications. However, patients with bilateral "Coats'" disease should be evaluated for systemic syndromes.

REFERENCES

Morris B, Foot B, Mulvihill A. A population-based study of Coats disease in the United Kingdom I: epidemiology and clinical features at diagnosis. *Eye (Lond)*. 2010;24(12):1797–1801.

Mulvihill A, Morris B. A population-based study of Coats disease in the United Kingdom II: investigation, treatment, and outcomes. *Eye (Lond)*. 2010; 24(12):1802–1807.

Shields JA, Shields CL, Honavar S, et al. Coats disease. Clinical variations and complications of Coats' disease in 150 cases. The 2000 Sanford Gifford Memorial Lecture. *Am J Ophthalmol*. 2001;131:561–571.

Shields JA, Shields CL, Honavar SG, et al. Classification and management of Coats disease. The 2000 Proctor lecture. *Am J Ophthalmol*. 2001;131:572–583.

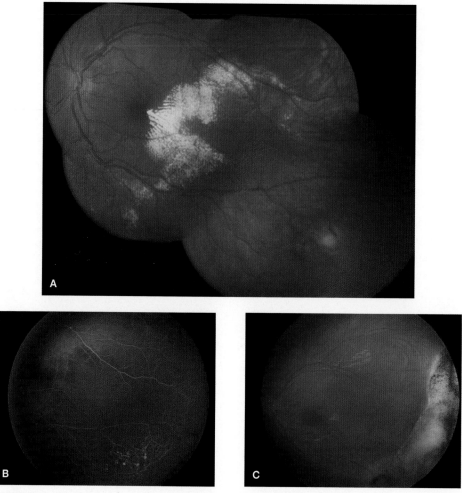

FIGURE 6-8. Coats' disease (stage 2) with mild temporal macular exudation (**A**) from telangiectatic vessels (**B**) that showed resolution after therapy (**C**) with cryotherapy and laser photocoagulation, allowing for good visual acuity.

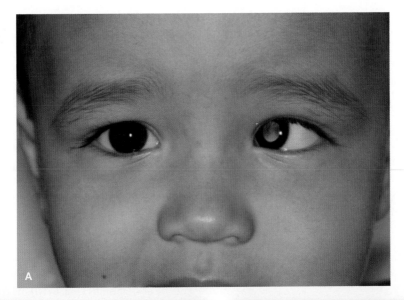

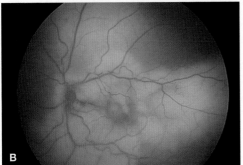

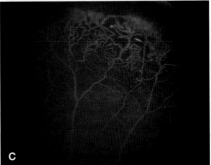

FIGURE 6-9. Coats' disease (stage 3) with xanthochroia (**A**) from massive subretinal exudation (**B**) and leaking retinal telangiectasia (**C**).

RETINOBLASTOMA

Carol L. Shields and Jerry A. Shields ▇

Retinoblastoma is the most common intra-ocular malignancy of children. It accounts for 4% of all childhood cancers. It is grouped into unilateral or bilateral involvement and subgrouped into sporadic or familial predisposition. This tumor manifests in young children, often within the first year of life. Worldwide, it is estimated that there are approximately 7202 children per year with retinoblastoma distributed in Asia excluding Japan (4027), Africa (1792), Latin America and the Caribbean (622), Europe (414), North America (258), Japan (59), and Oceania (21).

Etiology

• Retinoblastoma occurs in approximately 1 in 15,000 live births. Children with bilateral retinoblastoma are typically diagnosed around age 12 months, and those with unilateral retinoblastoma are typically diagnosed around 18 months. There is no race or gender predilection. Approximately two thirds of all cases are unilateral, and one third are bilateral.

• Retinoblastoma results from mutation of the retinoblastoma gene located on chromosome 13q14. In 1971, Knudson "two-hit" hypothesis for the development of retinoblastoma was proposed. In 1980, research confirmed that both alleles of retinoblastoma gene (*RB1*) at chromosome 13q14 locus were mutated in individuals with retinoblastoma. Currently, there are arguments that genomic instability and aneuploidy are likely responsible for the genesis of retinoblastoma.

• Bilateral and familial retinoblastoma arises from germline mutation in the retinoblastoma gene, but unilateral disease is more often a result of somatic mutation but can result from germline mutation in 15% of cases. Germline mutation retinoblastoma tends to be multifocal and can be associated with systemic cancers such as pinealoblastoma and remote cancers. A small subset of retinoblastoma patients display the 13q syndrome, which occurs from the mutation on chromosome 13 and involves features of microcephaly, a broad nasal bridge, hypertelorism, microphthalmos, epicanthus, ptosis, micrognathia, a short neck, low-set ears, facial asymmetry, anogenital malformations, hypoplastic thumbs and toes, and mental and psychomotor retardation.

Symptoms

• Retinoblastoma most often presents quietly with the painless development of leukocoria or strabismus (Fig. 6-10). It is most often discovered by the parents or grandparents more often than pediatricians.

• Occasionally, the child might have pain from secondary glaucoma that manifests in about 17% of patients. Rarely does the child complain of vision loss.

Signs

• The anterior segment classically displays leukocoria, and this feature is more prominent relative to tumor size. Neovascularization of the iris is occasionally found.

• Funduscopically, retinoblastoma appears as a solid, yellow-white tumor within the retina. It can appear with different growth patterns of intraretinal, subretinal (exophytic), vitreal (endophytic), and flat (diffuse). Small tumors appear intraretinal with a slightly dilated artery and vein. As the tumor enlarges, the vessels dilate and become slightly tortuous. Calcification can develop within the mass. Subretinal fluid, subretinal seeds, and vitreous seeds then develop. Occasionally, seeds can extend into the anterior chamber, producing a neoplastic pseudohypopyon. Advanced tumors lead to neovascularization of the iris with glaucoma, retinal neovascularization with vitreous hemorrhage, and invasion into the optic nerve and choroid.

Differential Diagnosis

- Retinal detachment from retinoblastoma can simulate:
    - Coats' disease
    - PHPV (PFV)
    - Toxocariasis
    - Retinal astrocytic hamartoma
    - Retinal astrocytoma
    - Combined hamartoma of the retina and RPE
    - Retinal detachment
    - FEVR
    - ROP
    - Incontinentia pigmenti
- Vitreous seeding from retinoblastoma can simulate:
    - Intraocular inflammation
    - Endophthalmitis
    - Vitreous hemorrhage
    - Leukemic infiltration
- Leukocoria from retinoblastoma can simulate:
    - Cataract
    - Glaucoma

Diagnostic Evaluation

- The diagnosis of retinoblastoma is established in the office setting using indirect ophthalmoscopy in the hands of an experienced examiner.
- Examination under anesthesia is reserved for detailed analysis of each eye, confirmation with diagnostic tests, and therapy.
- The tumor is confirmed on ultrasonography, showing it as a calcified dome-shaped mass.

- Fluorescein angiography will show intrinsic luxurious vascularity
- OCT will show subretinal fluid in cooperative children.
- CT will confirm the calcification within the mass, but most clinicians prefer MRI over CT because there is no radiation exposure with the former. MRI will show the enhancing intraocular mass and can be used to image the orbit and the brain, evaluating for optic nerve invasion and pinealoblastoma.
- Fine-needle aspiration biopsy should be avoided.
- Each affected eye is classified according to the International Classification of Retinoblastoma (Fig. 6-11):
    - Group A: retinoblastoma ≤3 mm
    - Group B: retinoblastoma >3 mm or in the macula or with clear subretinal fluid
    - Group C: retinoblastoma with subretinal or vitreous seeds ≤3 mm from tumor
    - Group D: retinoblastoma with subretinal or vitreous seeds >3 mm from tumor
    - Group E: extensive retinoblastoma filling >50% globe or with hemorrhage or iris neovascularization

Treatment

- Retinoblastoma management is complex and depends on many issues, including tumor laterality; macular involvement; tumor size; vitreous or subretinal seeding; relationship of the tumor to surrounding tissues, including the optic disc, choroid, iris, sclera, and orbit; general patient age and health; and the family's wishes. Laser photocoagulation, cryotherapy, thermotherapy, and plaque radiotherapy remain vitally important in the management of selective retinoblastoma. Enucleation, intravenous chemoreduction, intraarterial chemotherapy, and external-beam radiotherapy are used for more advanced retinoblastoma. External-beam radiotherapy is usually reserved s the last alternative treatment because of its numerous side effects and risks for late-onset cancers in children with germline mutations.

• Enucleation is used for advanced eyes, particularly unilateral tumors. After enucleation, the eye should be evaluated pathologically for high-risk features.

• Systemic intravenous chemoreduction is used for bilateral cases in which there are multiple tumors and often seeding (Fig. 6-12). Groups A, B, and C show greater than 90% success with chemoreduction, and group D shows about 50% success. Group E eyes are often enucleated.

• Intraarterial chemotherapy is showing promise for treatment of retinoblastoma as a primary treatment and after failure of other methods. In our preliminary experience, we have had 100% tumor control for groups C and D retinoblastoma and 33% control for group E (Fig. 6-13). Groups A and B retinoblastoma are not offered intraarterial chemotherapy yet because there are potentially profound risks such as cerebrovascular accident and ophthalmic artery obstruction.

• In rare instances, retinoblastoma can undergo spontaneous regression and show clinical features of complete tumor resolution without therapeutic intervention. Occasionally, this can lead to phthisis bulbi.

Prognosis

• Retinoblastoma is a highly malignant tumor with nearly 100% mortality if left untreated. In developed nations, most children present before high-risk features are found; thus, a good prognosis with lifesaving measures is achieved. In an analysis of

retinoblastoma worldwide, mortality paralleled the development of the nation.

• Histopathologic factors predict metastatic disease, including optic nerve invasion beyond the lamina cribrosa, massive choroidal invasion greater than 3 mm, scleral invasion, orbital invasion, and anterior chamber invasion. Some globes enucleated with retinoblastoma have high-risk features such as retrolaminar optic nerve invasion or massive uveal invasion of more than 3 mm. Patients with these features should receive additional chemotherapy.

• Children with germinal retinoblastoma have an increased risk of developing other primary malignancies over the course of their lifetimes. These tumors include principally intracranial retinoblastoma, osteogenic sarcoma of the long bones, and sarcoma of the soft tissues. The risk is estimated to be 30% by age 30 years, and the use of external-beam radiotherapy can increase the risk in the field of irradiation.

REFERENCES

Eagle RC Jr. High-risk features and tumor differentiation in retinoblastoma: a retrospective histopathologic study. *Arch Pathol Lab Med.* 2009;133:1203–1209.

Kivela T. The epidemiological challenge of the most frequent eye cancer: retinoblastoma, an issue of birth and death. *Br J Ophthalmol.* 2009;93:1129–1131.

Shields CL, Shields JA. Basic understanding of current classification and management of retinoblastoma. *Curr Opin Ophthalmol.* 2006;17:228–234.

Shields JA, Shields CL. Retinoblastoma. In Shields JA, Shields CL, eds. *Atlas of Intraocular Tumors.* Philadelphia: Lippincott Williams & Wilkins; 2008: 293–365.

Shields CL, Shields JA. Retinoblastoma management: advances in enucleation, intravenous chemoreduction, and intra-arterial chemotherapy. *Curr Opin Ophthalmol.* 2010;21:203–212.

Wong FL, Boice JD Jr, Abramson DH, et al. Cancer incidence after retinoblastoma. Radiation dose and sarcoma risk. *JAMA.* 1997;278:1262–1267.

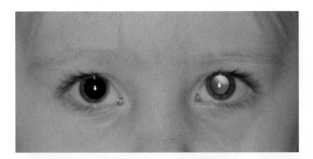

FIGURE 6-10. Leukocoria (left eye) from retinoblastoma.

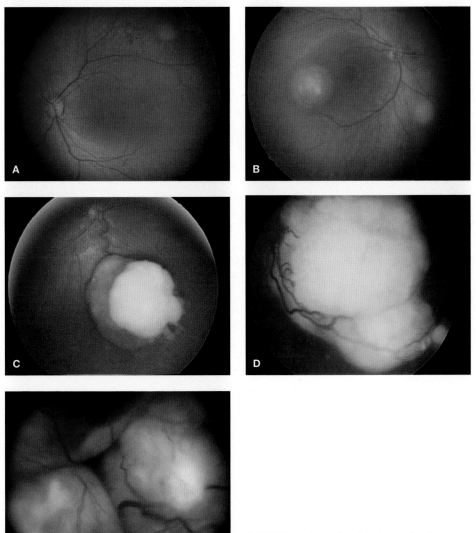

FIGURE 6-11. Examples of the international classification of retinoblastoma into groups A, B, C, D, and E.

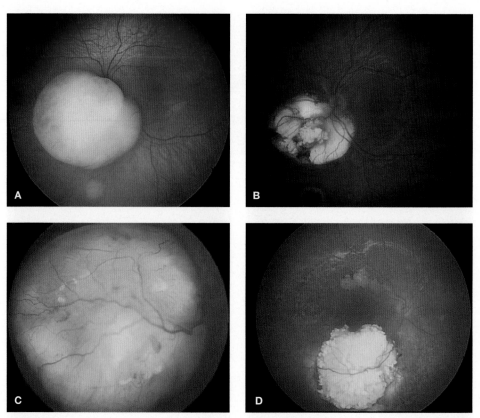

FIGURE 6-12. Response of retinoblastoma to intravenous chemoreduction in two cases showing before therapy (**A, C**) and after therapy (**B, D**).

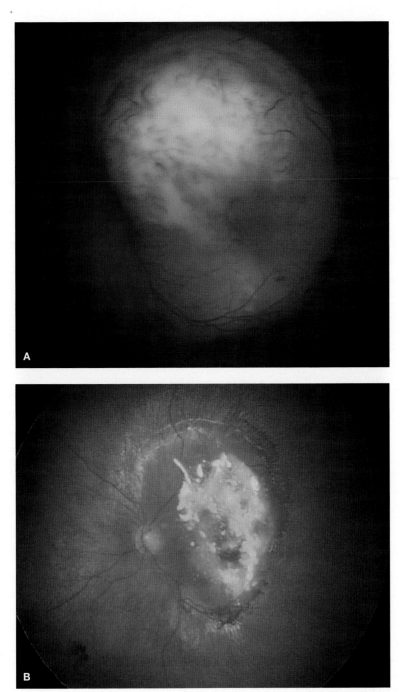

FIGURE 6-13. Response of retinoblastoma to intra-arterial chemotherapy showing before therapy (**A**) and after therapy (**B**).

CONGENITAL HYPERTROPHY OF THE RETINAL PIGMENT EPITHELIUM

Anuradha Ganesh and Alex V. Levin

Congenital hypertrophy of the RPE (CHRPE) is a benign, asymptomatic condition consisting of one or more well-demarcated, pigmented, flat, nonmitotic lesions at the level of the RPE.

Epidemiology and Etiology

- Solitary CHRPE occurs in approximately 1 in 60 in the general population. No racial predilection has been reported.

- Histopathologically, the lesion consists of a focal area in which the RPE cells are taller and more densely packed with melanosomes. The individual melanosomes are larger and more spherical compared with those of the normal RPE. The associated depigmented lacunae, halos, or "tails" correspond to areas where the melanosomes are sparser.

History

- Patients are usually asymptomatic. Often, the disorder is noted as an incidental finding during ophthalmoscopy.

Signs

CHRPE may take one of two forms:

- *Solitary:* This is the most common form. It is characteristically a unilateral, deeply pigmented, flat, circular lesion with a well-circumscribed margin. These may be pinpoint or two or three disc diameters in size. The lesion may be solid black with a marginal halo of hypopigmentation. Depigmented lacunae may be seen within the lesion.

- *Multiple:* Multifocal CHRPE lesions are seen in more than 80% of patients with familial adenomatous polyposis (FAP) or Gardner's syndrome, a familial condition of colonic polyps and extraintestinal osteomas and fibromas with uniform progression to colonic cancer if not treated. The lesions are bilateral, multiple, and scattered and more often have a "cometoid" configuration with a hypopigmented tail on the side of the lesion closer to the macula (**Fig. 6-14**).

Differential Diagnosis

- Choroidal melanoma
- Choroidal nevus
- Combined hamartoma of the retina and RPE
- Reactive hyperplasia of the RPE (e.g., posttraumatic)
- Bear tracks
- Chorioretinal scars (e.g., toxoplasmosis, congenital varicella)

Diagnostic Evaluation

- The characteristic appearance of CHRPE should enable the clinician to make the diagnosis and differentiate it from other lesions. Fluorescein angiography reveals hypofluorescence throughout all phases of the angiogram except in the region of the haloes and lacunae, which show transmission hyperfluorescence. The lesions are not associated with subretinal fluid or orange pigment.

Treatment and Prognosis

- Although overlying photoreceptor loss and alterations of the RPE may lead to visual field defects, CHRPEs are usually benign and asymptomatic and do not affect visual acuity or visual field.

- Over time, subtle enlargement of the lesions and development of an elevated nodule representing adenoma or adenocarcinoma has rarely been reported. Hence, they should be observed periodically for growth.

- Patients with bilateral or multiple unilateral lesions suggestive of those seen in FAP or Gardner's syndrome should be referred for periodic colonoscopy usually beginning at 7 or 8 years old.

REFERENCES

Shields JA, Eagle RC Jr, Shields CL, et al. Malignant transformation of congenital hypertrophy of the retinal pigment epithelium. *Ophthalmology.* 2009;116:2213–2216.

Shields JA, Shields CL. Tumors and related lesions of the pigment epithelium. In: Shields JA, Shields CL, eds. *Intraocular Tumors. A Text and Atlas.* Philadelphia: WB Saunders; 1992:437–460.

Traboulsi EI. Ocular manifestations of familial adenomatous polyposis (Gardner syndrome). *Ophthalmol Clin North Am.* 2005;18:163–166.

Traboulsi EI, Maumenee IH, Krush AJ, et al. Congenital hypertrophy of the retinal pigment epithelium predicts colorectal polyposis in Gardner's syndrome. *Arch Ophthalmol.* 1990;108:525–526.

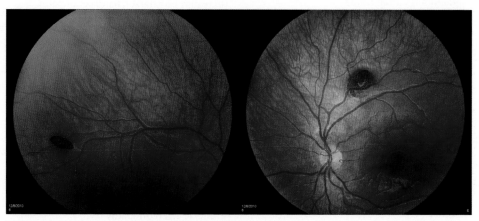

FIGURE 6-14. Congenital hypertrophy of the retinal pigment epithelium. Fundus photograph of both eyes shows bilateral hyperpigmented retinal lesions in a patient with Gardner's syndrome. The lesion in the right eye has a "cometoid" appearance with a hypopigmented tail on the side of the lesion closer to the macula. The lesions in both eyes show a marginal halo of depigmentation.

FAMILIAL EXUDATIVE VITREORETINOPATHY

Anuradha Ganesh and Alex V. Levin ◼

FEVR is a hereditary vitreoretinal disorder characterized by failure of peripheral retinal vascularization and resulting secondary complications such as neovascularization, retinal folds, traction, and detachment.

Epidemiology and Etiology

● FEVR is a rare disorder. The prevalence has not been calculated. Ninety percent of affected individuals may be asymptomatic.

● FEVR is genetically heterogeneous and is associated with mutations in the *FZD4* (autosomal dominant FEVR), *LRP5* (autosomal dominant and recessive FEVR), *NDP* (X linked recessive FEVR), and *TSPAN12* (autosomal dominant FEVR) genes. Autosomal dominant inheritance is the most common mode of inheritance.

History

● The clinical appearance of FEVR varies considerably, even within families, with severely affected patients often registered as blind during infancy and mildly affected patients having few or no visual problems.

● Infants may present with strabismus or leukocoria caused by retinal detachment.

● There is no association with prematurity or oxygen exposure.

Signs

● Infants born with FEVR are otherwise healthy. Ophthalmic findings are frequently asymmetric and highly variable. The classic finding in FEVR is peripheral retinal capillary nonperfusion (Fig. 6-15). Usually, the avascular zone is confined to the temporal periphery, but it may extend for 360 degrees.

● The disease may not progress further or may lead to peripheral neovascularization at the border of posterior vascularized and anterior avascular retina (Fig. 6-16). Retinal fold; peripheral fibrovascular mass; vitreous hemorrhage; and progression to even more severe changes such as tractional, exudative, and even rhegmatogenous retinal detachment may occur. Intraretinal and subretinal exudation may be associated.

● In severe cases with retinal detachment, there may be cataract, band keratopathy, neovascular glaucoma, or phthisis.

● Asymptomatic individuals may manifest regions of peripheral avascularity with abnormal vascular anastomoses visible clinically or only on intravenous fluorescein angiography.

Differential Diagnosis

● ROP

● Incontinentia pigmenti

● Coats' disease

● PFV

● Sickle cell retinopathy

● Other causes of infantile retinal nonattachment or detachment

Diagnostic Evaluation

● The diagnosis of FEVR is based on a family history compatible with autosomal dominant, autosomal recessive or X-linked recessive inheritance, and bilateral peripheral retinal avascularity.

● If FEVR is suspected, examination of the peripheral retina of asymptomatic family members may also reveal findings consistent with the diagnosis. Tests that may help in confirming the diagnosis include fluorescein angiography (abrupt cessation of peripheral retinal capillary network, and possible abnormal vasculature) and genetic testing.

Treatment and Prognosis

- Laser photocoagulation to the peripheral avascular retina and neovascularization may prevent progression of fibrovascular complications.

- The value of prophylactic treatment is controversial, and most authors suggest treatment only if neovascularization is present. Prevention of retinal detachment is far more effective than treatment after detachment occurs.

- FEVR is a lifelong disease, and events such as neovascularization, retinal detachments, and vitreous hemorrhage may occur at any age. Perinatal screening continued for several years is advisable in at-risk individuals.

REFERENCES

Robitaille JM, Zheng B, Wallace K, et al. The role of Frizzled-4 mutations in familial exudative vitreoretinopathy and Coats disease. *Br J Ophthalmol.* 2010; 95(4):574–579.

Shukla D, Singh J, Sudheer G, et al. Familial exudative vitreoretinopathy (FEVR). Clinical profile and management. *Indian J Ophthalmol.* 2003;51:323–328.

Toomes C, Downey L. Familial exudative vitreoretinopathy, autosomal dominant. In: Pagon RA, Bird TC, Dolan CR, et al, eds. *GeneReviews.* Seattle: University of Washington; 2008.

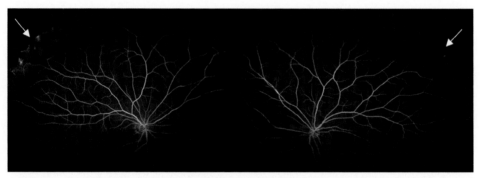

FIGURE 6-15. Familial exudative vitreoretinopathy. Fundus fluorescein angiogram clearly demonstrates bilateral peripheral retinal capillary nonperfusion and leakage (*arrows*).

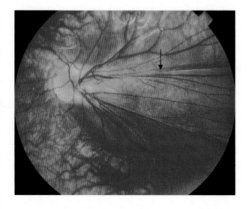

FIGURE 6-16. Familial exudative vitreoretinopathy. Retinal tractional fold (*arrow*) causing straightening of vessels at the disc.

PERSISTENT FETAL VASCULATURE

Alok S. Bansal ▪

PFV, formerly referred to as PHPV, is a developmental malformation of the eye that results from failure of regression of the primary vitreal hyaloidal vessels and other associated vessels in the tunica vasculosa lentis, iris, or both.

PFV is most often unilateral and nonheritable. When bilateral (10%), there is more often systemic associations and the potential for a genetic basis (**Table 6-3**).

Signs

• There are many forms of PFV, ranging in a spectrum from anterior findings to posterior findings.

• Isolated anterior PFV (**Fig. 6-17A**) is characterized by a retrolental vascularized membrane, variable degree of cataract, drawn-in ciliary processes (**Fig. 6-17B**), traction on the peripheral retina caused by a membranous transformation of the anterior vitreous face, shallow anterior chamber, poor pupil dilation, and microphthalmos.

• The more severe posterior PFV is characterized by a stalk of tissue extending from the optic nerve to the retrolental area, a retinal fold

with or without tractional retinal detachment (**Fig. 6-17C**), macular pigmentary disruption, and variable degrees of optic nerve dysplasia. The lens can be clear in isolated posterior PFV.

Differential Diagnosis

• Norrie's disease
• Coats' disease
• Toxocariasis
• ROP
• FEVR
• Incontinentia pigmenti
• Retinal dysplasia
• Retinal detachment (overt or covert trauma)

Diagnostic Evaluation

• The diagnosis of PFV can be made with careful ophthalmoscopic examination. Depending on the age of the child, an examination under anesthesia may be considered.

• If significant media opacity precludes a view of the fundus, B-scan ultrasonography may demonstrate a stalk or retinal detachment. Careful examination of the iris may reveal anterior signs of persistent vasculature.

Treatment

• The goals of management include clearing the media opacity to allow visual development and prevent complications of

TABLE 6-3. Systemic and Genetic Basis of Ocular Disorders

Syndrome	Inheritance	Chromosome	Gene	Function
Wagner's	AD	5q14.3	CSPG2	Binds to hyaluronan in vitreous
Knobloch's	AR	21q22.3	COL18A1	Cleaves to endostatin
PFV	AR	10q11-21	Not known	
PFV	XLR	Xp11.4	NDP	Signaling pathways for morphogenesis
ASMD	AD	10q22.3-25	PITX3	Regulates ocular morphogenesis

AD, autosomal dominant; AR, autosomal recessive; ASMD, anterior segment mesenchymal dysgenesis; CSPG, chondroitin sulfate proteoglycan; COL18A1, collagen type 18 alpha 1; NDP, Norrie disease pseudoglioma; PFV, persistent fetal vasculature; PITX3, paired like homeo domain 3.

untreated PFV such as glaucoma and retinal detachment.

- Either anterior limbal or pars plana approaches to lensectomy, membranectomy, and vitrectomy may be used.

- Aggressive amblyopia treatment with aphakic contact lenses are required to achieve optimum vision. The prognosis for patients with pure anterior PFV is better than for those with posterior PFV.

REFERENCES

Goldberg MF. Persistent fetal vasculature (PFV): an integrated interpretation of signs and symptoms associated with persistent hyperplastic primary vitreous (PHPV). LIV Edward Jackson Memorial Lecture. *Am J Ophthalmol.* 1997;124(5):587–626.

Pollard ZF. Persistent hyperplastic primary vitreous: diagnosis, treatment, and results. *Trans Am Ophthalmol Soc.* 1997;95:487–549.

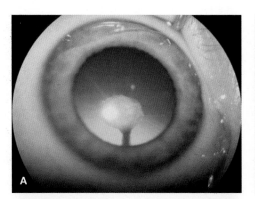

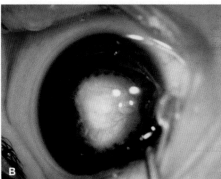

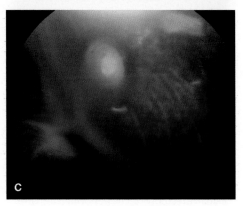

FIGURE 6-17. Persistent fetal vasculature (PFV). **A.** The retrolental stalk is attributable to failure of regression of the primary vitreal hyaloidal vessels. **B.** PFV demonstrating a vascularized retrolental membrane, cataract, and drawn-in ciliary processes. **C.** PFV demonstrating a retinal fold with an associated tractional retinal detachment.

JUVENILE RETINOSCHISIS

Barry N. Wasserman ■

Etiology

● An X-linked inherited disease, juvenile retinoschisis is the most common cause of macular degeneration in young boys.

● Mutation of the *XLRS1* gene results in retinal dysfunction caused by splitting of the retinal layers and the characteristic inner retinal layer schisis and stellate maculopathy.

Symptoms

● Patients may present with mildly reduced vision that may deteriorate to less than 20/400, although one study suggested no significant disease progression in children over an average of 12 years of follow-up.

● Visual loss is attributable to foveal schisis or retinal detachment.

Signs

● Fundus examination reveals foveal schisis in a stellate pattern. In approximately 50% of patients, peripheral retinoschisis of the nerve fiber layer occurs with inner layer holes and possible progression to full-thickness retinal detachment.

● Whitish dots or patches in the retinal mid-periphery and periphery (snowflakes) may be seen and are thought to represent abnormal Muller cell footplates.

● Pigmented demarcation lines indicate prior full-thickness detachment.

● Spontaneous vitreous hemorrhage results from vessels bridging the inner retinal layer holes.

Differential Diagnosis

● Nicotinic acid maculopathy

● Rhegmatogenous retinal detachment

● Goldman-Favre disease

● Wagner's vitreoretinal dystrophy and other vitreoretinopathies

● Cystoid macular edema

● Norrie's disease

Diagnostic Evaluation

● Characteristic family history of affected males with intervening unaffected female carriers

● Fundus examination reveals stellate appearance in fovea, which resembles cystoid macular edema (Fig. 6-18).

● Fluorescein angiography does not show leakage.

● Retinal pigment epithelial pigmentary changes and vitreous veils are seen.

● Ocular coherence tomography may demonstrate schisis extending into the retinal periphery (Fig. 6-19).

● Electroretinogram reveals diminished B-wave amplitudes, but electro-oculogram results are normal.

Treatment

● Genetic counseling is recommended for families with X-linked juvenile retinoschisis.

● Some patients with cystoid macular changes have shown improvement in visual acuity and OCT finding when treated with topical or oral carbonic anhydrase inhibitors.

● Prophylactic laser photocoagulation is not recommended and can lead to retinal detachment.

● Surgery using scleral buckling and pars plana vitrectomy can be performed for vitreous hemorrhage and retinal detachment.

Prognosis

● Some patients maintain good vision into adulthood, but visual acuity commonly deteriorates, particularly when peripheral retinal schisis is present.

REFERENCES

Apushkin MA, Fishman GA. Use of dorzolamide for patients with X-linked retinoschisis. *Retina.* 2006;26:741–745.

Goodwin P. Hereditary retinal disease. *Curr Opin Ophthalmol.* 2008;19:255–262.

Kjellström S, Vijayasarathy C, Ponjavic V, et al. Long-term 12 year follow-up of X-linked congenital retinoschisis. *Ophthalmic Genet.* 2010;31(3):114–125.

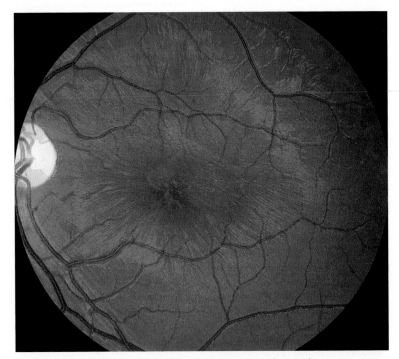

FIGURE 6-18. Juvenile X-linked retinoschisis with cystic appearance in the macula.

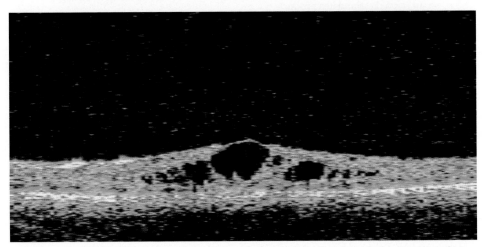

FIGURE 6-19. Juvenile X-linked retinoschisis. Ocular coherence tomography of macula demonstrating schisis cavities.

RETINOPATHY OF PREMATURITY

Anuradha Ganesh and Barry N. Wasserman ■

ROP is a proliferative retinopathy of premature, low-birthweight infants.

Epidemiology and Etiology

• Each year, ROP is believed to affect an estimated 14,000 to 16,000 premature, low-birthweight infants in the United States.

• The majority of infants who develop ROP undergo spontaneous regression (85%). The rest develop threshold ROP requiring treatment, and 6% to 7% of infants become legally blind despite treatment. Infants born before 32 weeks gestation or those with a birthweight of less than 1500 g who have received oxygen therapy are at risk.

• In preterm infants, retinal vascular development is incomplete. Instead of continued progression from the optic nerve head anteriorly along the plane of retina, vascular migrations ceases, leading to an area of avascular retina. The extent of avascular retina depends mainly on the degree of prematurity at birth. The resultant hypoxia stimulates production of substances such as vascular endothelial growth factor (VEGF), which trigger neovascularization, known as extraretinal fibrovascular proliferation (ERFP), off the surface of the retina. ERFP may lead to hemorrhage and contraction, with resultant retinal detachment. In many cases, the retinopathy abnormalities spontaneously regress without treatment.

History

• Infants are considered high risk and are screened for ROP if their birthweight is less than 1500 g or gestational age is 32 weeks or less. Selected infants with an unstable clinical course, including those requiring cardiorespiratory support, with birthweights between 1500 and 2000 g or gestational age of more than 32 weeks may also be screened at the discretion of the neonatologist.

Signs

• The International Classification of ROP (ICROP) categorizes ROP by location, called the zone, or by severity, called the stage.

• In addition, the presence or absence of *"plus" disease* is evaluated (**Table 6-4, Fig. 6-20**). An eye has *"plus" disease* when there are at least two quadrants of dilation of veins and tortuosity of arterioles in the posterior pole (**Fig. 6-20C**). Iris engorgement, pupillary rigidity, vitreous haze, or

TABLE 6-4. International Classification of Retinopathy of Prematurity

Location	
Zone I	Posterior circle of retina centered on the optic nerve with a radius of twice the disc-fovea distance.
Zone II	Circular area of retina from the edge of zone I to the nasal ora serrata
Zone III	Remaining temporal crescent of retina
Extent	
Number of clock hours or 30-degree sectors involved	
Severity	
Stage 1	Demarcation line at the junction of posterior vascularized and anterior avascular retina
Stage 2	Ridge (demarcation line with volume)
Stage 3	Ridge with ERFP
Stage 4	Subtotal retinal detachment
Stage 4A	Extrafoveal
Stage 4B	Fovea is detached
Stage 5	Total retinal detachment with funnel

ERFP, extraretinal fibrovascular proliferation.

retinal hemorrhages are often seen in "plus" disease. *"Plus" disease* denotes increased severity. *Pre-plus disease* refers to more mild posterior pole vascular dilation and tortuosity but insufficient for diagnosis of plus disease.

- "Popcorn" lesions are named so because of their similarity to kernels of white fluffy popcorn floating above the developed retina. They represent buds of vascular proliferation behind the ridge or demarcation line. Popcorn lesions are only significant when they are part of active ERFP. Vitreous hemorrhage and preretinal hemorrhage can occasionally be seen in eyes with severe ERFP.

- In *acute posterior ROP (AP-ROP)*, vascularization is only present in zone I and there is plus disease. This subtype of ROP, previously termed "rush" disease, is associated with an aggressive course and a risk for rapid progression into stage 4 or 5.

- After treatment of threshold ROP, most will regress by a process of involution or cicatrization, often yielding good visual acuity. This may be accompanied by a broad range of sequelae such as failure of peripheral retinal vascularization, abnormal branching of retinal vessels, retinal pigmentary changes, vitreoretinal interface changes, retinal folds, and distortion and ectopia of the macula.

- The characteristic findings of ROP are present in the setting of infants born prematurely of low birthweight with a history of oxygen exposure and other disorders associated with prematurity such as sepsis, intraventricular hemorrhage, anemia, or feeding difficulties.

Differential Diagnosis

Differential diagnosis depends on the stage of the disease.

- In less severe ROP, conditions that cause peripheral retinal vascular changes and retinal dragging should be considered:
  - Incontinentia pigmenti
  - FEVR
  - PFV
  - Other causes of infantile retinal nonattachment or detachment

- In advanced cicatricial ROP, the differential diagnosis is consistent with retinal detachment or leukocoria:
  - Retinoblastoma
  - Cataract
  - Coats' disease
  - Toxocariasis

Diagnostic Evaluation

- Careful examination of neonates with indirect ophthalmoscopy in the intensive care unit or at discharge is recommended between 4 and 6 weeks of chronologic (postnatal) age or, alternatively, within the 31st to 33rd week of postconceptional or postmenstrual age (gestational age at birth plus chronologic age), whichever is later.

- Digital imaging is a useful adjunct during fundus examinations.

Treatment and Prognosis

- The purpose of screening for ROP is to identify infants with advanced ROP who would progress to retinal detachment unless treated. *"Threshold" disease* (a level of ROP at which there is a 50% chance of progression to retinal detachment without treatment) is characterized by five contiguous clock hours of ERFP with plus disease. *"Prethreshold" disease* is defined as any zone I-stage of ROP or zone II-stage 2 + ROP/stage 3 ROP/stage 3 + ROP but less extensive than threshold disease. The Early Treatment for ROP (ET-ROP) study divided prethreshold eyes into two groups

TABLE 6-5. Early Treatment Retinopathy or Prematurity Prethreshold Types

Type I
Zone I: any stage ROP with plus disease
Zone I: stage 3 ROP without plus disease
Zone II: stage 2 or 3 ROP with plus disease

Type II
Zone I: stage 1 or 2 ROP without plus disease
Zone II: stage 3 ROP without plus disease

ROP, retinopathy of prematurity.

(Table 6-5) and recommended that peripheral retinal ablation be applied to any eye with type 1 prethreshold ROP.

- Peripheral retinal ablation of the anterior avascular zone may be performed with cryotherapy or laser photocoagulation. The latter, delivered with an indirect ophthalmoscope, has replaced cryotherapy for threshold ROP (Fig. 6-21). Better visual outcomes have been achieved with laser treatment. More advanced stages of ROP (stages 4 and 5) require scleral buckling, vitrectomy, or both. The prognosis for visual recovery after retinal detachment remains poor.

- Despite appropriate screening and timing of intervention, ROP continues to progress in some babies. This has led to research into newer and more effective modalities of therapy. Ongoing studies evaluating the efficacy and safety of intravitreal injections of anti-VEGF drug bevacizumab (Avastin) for ROP suggest that this therapeutic modality may produce similar or better outcomes than laser photocoagulation.

REFERENCES

Davitt BV, Wallace DK. Plus disease. *Surv Ophthalmol.* 2009;54:663–670.

Kemper AR, Wallace DK, Quinn GE. Systematic review of digital imaging screening strategies for retinopathy of prematurity. *Pediatrics.* 2008;122:825–830.

Mintz-Hittner HA, Kuffel RR Jr. Intravitreal injection of bevacizumab (Avastin) for treatment of stage 3 retinopathy of prematurity in zone I or posterior zone II. *Retina.* 2008;28:831–838.

Reynolds JD. Retinopathy of prematurity. *Int Ophthalmol Clin.* 2010;50:1–13.

Section on Ophthalmology American Academy of Pediatrics; American Academy of Ophthalmology; American Association for Pediatric Ophthalmology and Strabismus. Screening examination of premature infants for retinopathy of prematurity. *Pediatrics.* 2006;117(2):572–576.

Vander JF, McNamara JA, Tasman W, et al. Revised indications for early treatment of retinopathy of prematurity. *Arch Ophthalmol.* 2005;123:406–407.

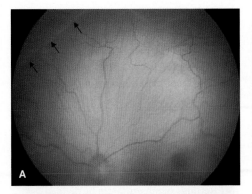

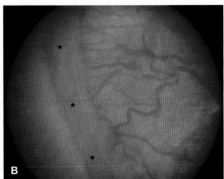

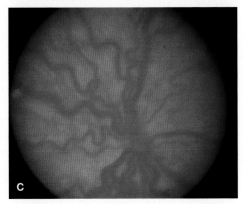

FIGURE 6-20. Retinopathy of prematurity. **A.** Zone II, stage II disease with mild to moderate "plus" disease. At the superior aspect of the retina, the vessel development has ceased, and a white ridge (*arrows*) is seen. Avascular, undeveloped retina is seen beyond the ridge. (Courtesy of Sharon Lehman, MD.) **B.** Zone II, stage III disease with "plus" disease. Neovascularization is seen rising into the vitreous above the ridge (*asterisks*). (Courtesy of William Tasman, MD.) **C.** "Plus" disease with severe vascular dilation and tortuosity. (Courtesy of William Tasman, MD.)

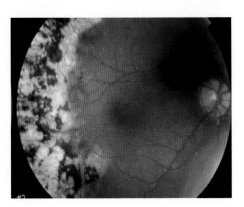

FIGURE 6-21. Retinopathy of prematurity after successful treatment with laser photocoagulation and peripheral chorioretinal scars. (Courtesy of William Tasman, MD.)

RETINITIS PIGMENTOSA

Barry N. Wasserman ▦

Etiology

● Retinitis pigmentosa is a group of diseases characterized by night blindness (nyctalopia); slow, painless, progressive peripheral visual field loss; and progressive deterioration of the electroretinogram.

● Virtually every inheritance pattern has been reported, and more than 70 genes have been shown to be causative when mutated. Phenotypic and genetic heterogeneity are common.

● The common pathway is retinal receptor cell death via apoptosis.

● Retinitis pigmentosa may be found in isolation or in association with systemic or neurodegenerative disease.

Symptoms

● Retinitis pigmentosa begins in childhood, adolescence, or early adulthood with nyctalopia and issues of light to dark adaptation.

● Patients may also complain of loss of peripheral vision.

● Other symptoms may include photophobia, variable visual acuity, and unusual colors in visual perception.

Signs

● Visual acuity may range from 20/20 to no light perception but is usually preserved early in the disease.

● Visual field constriction is progressive.

● Posterior subcapsular cataracts are common in adult patients.

● Retinal findings may be minimal in children, but eventually, classic "bone spicule" pattern of midperipheral hyperpigmentation occurs, with associated arteriolar thinning

and waxy pallor of the optic nerve (**Fig. 6-22**).

● Other macular changes, including loss of foveal reflex, irregularities of the internal limiting membrane, and cystoid maculopathy, can occur.

● Electroretinogram findings progress to nondetectable.

Differential Diagnosis

● Retinitis pigmentosa can be divided into nonsyndromic and syndromic types. Nonsyndromic types include the autosomal dominant and recessive forms, as well as X-linked forms. Rare mitochondrial DNA mutation types also occur.

● Syndromic types of retinitis pigmentosa are extremely varied and include:

▪ Syndromes associated with deafness, most commonly Usher's syndrome

▪ Syndromes associated with metabolic diseases, including Abetalipoproteinemia (Bassen-Kornzweig disease); Zellweger's syndrome (cerebrohepatorenal syndrome); Refsum's disease; mucopolysaccharidoses types I, II, III; and neuronal ceroid lipofuscinosis (Batten's disease)

▪ Kearns-Sayre syndrome

▪ Syndromes with renal associations, including Fanconi's syndrome, cystinosis, Senior-Loken syndrome

▪ Dysmorphic syndromes, including Cohen's syndrome, Jeune's syndrome, Cockayne's syndrome

▪ Pigmentary retinopathies: pseudoretinitis pigmentosa

▪ Cancer-associated retinopathy

▪ Congenital infections, including syphilis, rubella, and CMV

▪ Drug-associated retinopathy, including phenothiazines and chloroquine

▪ Retinal vascular occlusion

Diagnostic Evaluation

- Ocular examination may show classic findings but findings may be normal early in the disease.

- Visual field testing reveals constriction, and electroretinogram shows that rod and cone signals are depressed or extinguished. Contrast sensitivity is sometimes decreased.

- Genetic testing maybe helpful for determining subtypes and prognosis.

Treatment

- Genetic counseling is advised.

- The use of vitamin A is controversial.

- Oral or topical carbonic anhydrase inhibitors can be helpful for patients who have associated macular edema.

- Cataract extraction should be performed when indicated but may have a higher risk of postoperative cystoid macular edema.

- Gene therapy is under investigation.

- Retinal pigment epithelial transplant and electronic retinal implants are also under investigation.

- Low vision services are recommended as the disease progresses.

Prognosis

- Visual acuity may remain better than 20/40 in more than half of patients in their 40s. However, 25% may have less than 20/200 and are considered legally blind. Only 1 in every 1000 patients develops no light perception.

- Whereas individuals with X-linked types may have the worst visual acuity prognosis, those with sector type autosomal dominant retinitis pigmentosa generally retain good vision.

REFERENCES

Hamel C. Retinitis pigmentosa. *Orphanet J Rare Dis.* 2006;1:40.

Goodwin P. Hereditary retinal disease. *Curr Opin Ophthalmol.* 2008;19:255–262.

Grover S, Fishman GA, Anderson RJ, et al. Visual acuity impairment in patients with retinitis pigmentosa at age 45 years or older. *Ophthalmology.* 1999; 106(9):1780–1785.

Jackson H, Garway-Heath D, Rosen P, et al. Outcome of cataract surgery in patients with retinitis pigmentosa. *Br J Ophthalmol.* 2001;85(8):936–938.

Jacobson SG, Cideciyan AV. Treatment possibilities for retinitis pigmentosa. *N Engl J Med.* 2010;363:1669–1671.

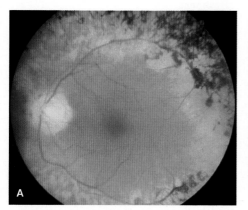 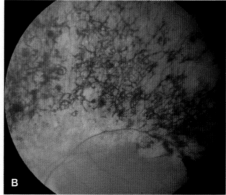

FIGURE 6-22. A. Retinitis pigmentosa fundus photo demonstrating optic nerve waxy pallor, vascular attenuation, and midperipheral "bone spicule" pigmentary retinopathy. **B.** Higher magnification photograph of midperipheral "bone spicule" retinopathy.

MYELINATED NERVE FIBERS

Barry N. Wasserman ■

Etiology

● Whitish sheets or patches of myelin distributed along portions of the nerve fiber layer of the retina. Usually unilateral, myelin is produced by oligodendrocytes and is normal along the optic nerve but does not normally progress beyond the lamina cribrosa.

● Ectopic oligodendrocytes are associated with myelin in the retinal nerve fiber layer, generally near the optic nerve.

● Myelinated nerve fibers may be found in 1% of eyes and may be an isolated finding or may be associated with other abnormalities, including neurofibromatosis and Gorlin's syndrome.

Symptoms

● May be asymptomatic but sometimes associated with high axial myopia and amblyopia in the affected eye

Signs

● Poor vision on examination associated with feathery grey-white patches along the retinal nerve fiber layer. They are often found at the optic nerve and along the vascular arcades, more commonly superiorly (Fig. 6-23A).

● There may also be a patch unconnected to the optic nerve (Fig. 6-23B).

● High myopic astigmatism with anisometropic amblyopia is reported.

● If extensive, myelinated nerve fibers can cause leukocoria (Fig. 6-24).

Differential Diagnosis

● Branch retinal artery occlusion

● Cotton wool patches

● When extensive, myelinated nerve fibers can yield leukocoria, in which case the following must be ruled out:
  ■ Retinoblastoma
  ■ Coats' disease
  ■ Coloboma
  ■ Cataract
  ■ ROP
  ■ PFV
  ■ FEVR

Diagnostic Evaluation

● Myelinated nerve fibers are diagnosed by clinical fundus examination. Feathery grey-white patches are noted superficially in the nerve fiber layer along the vascular arcades, often in close proximity to the optic disc.

● Visual field testing may reveal absolute or relative scotomas corresponding to the myelinated fibers.

● Spectral domain OCT has shown normal morphology of the fovea, suggesting that amblyopia may be more related to anisometropia than to an anatomic abnormality.

Treatment

● No treatment is needed for asymptomatic myelinated nerve fibers.

● When associated with anisometropic amblyopia, appropriate aggressive amblyopia treatment should be instituted.

Prognosis

● When dense amblyopia is associated with myelinated nerve fibers, the prognosis is variable and guarded.

● Outcomes are worse when associated with high myopia and history of associated strabismus.

REFERENCES

Gharai S, Prakash G, Kumar DA, et al. Spectral domain optical coherence tomographic characteristics of unilateral peripapillary myelinated retinal nerve fibers involving the macula. *J AAPOS.* 2010;14: 432–434.

Lee MS, Gonzalez C. Unilateral peripapillary myelinated retinal nerve fibers associated with strabismus, amblyopia, and myopia. *Am J Ophthalmol.* 1998;125:554–556.

Tarabishy AB, Alexandrou TJ, Traboulsi EI. Syndrome of myelinated retinal nerve fibers, myopia, and amblyopia: a review. *Surv Ophthalmol.* 2007;52:588–596.

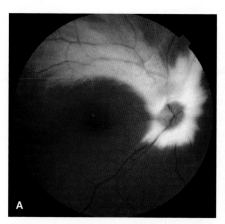
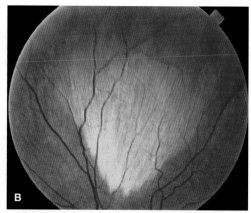

FIGURE 6-23. Myelinated nerve fibers. **A.** Fundus photograph with extensive feathery white myelination extending in all directions from the optic nerve. **B.** Myelinated nerve fibers superior to the optic nerve without direct connection to the optic nerve. (Courtesy of William Tasman, MD.)

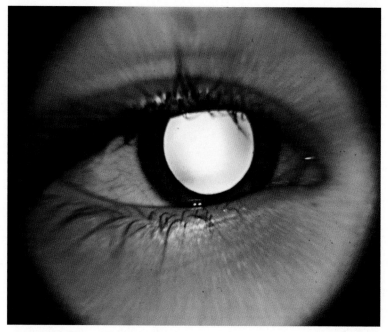

FIGURE 6-24. Leukocoria in a patient with extensive myelinated nerve fibers. (Courtesy of William Tasman, MD.)

STARGARDT'S DISEASE OR FUNDUS FLAVIMACULATA

Barry N. Wasserman ■

Etiology

● A largely autosomal recessively inherited atrophic macular dystrophy, Stargardt's disease is associated with mutations of the *ABCA4* gene on chromosome 1p. Specific mutations have not been correlated with electroretinographic characteristics or fundus appearance. This gene may also act as a modifier gene in other retinal dystrophies with other known gene mutations.

● Lipofuscin accumulation in the RPE is associated with vision loss.

● Other types of Stargardt's disease include autosomal dominant phenotypes associated with mutations in the genes *ELOVL4* or *PROM1* and mitochondrial phenocopies.

Symptoms

● Decreased central visual acuity is usually acute and precipitous in the first or second decade of life. Vision loss is sometimes seen in absence of ophthalmoscopic findings.

● Painless, progressive, slow visual deterioration to the 20/200 range may occur through the third decade of life.

Signs

● Visual acuity is decreased to varying degrees at presentation. Fundus examination results may be normal or only show a loss of foveal reflex early in the disease, but later, yellow subretinal "flecks" are seen (Fig. 6-25). Classically, the flecks are found centrally in Stargardt's disease, with more profound and progressive vision loss, and in the midperiphery in fundus flavimaculata, with better vision prognosis. Flecks have been described as "fish-scale shaped" and hence the name "pisciform." Eventually, the macula takes on a beaten bronze appearance and sometimes a bull's eye maculopathy.

● Fluorescein angiography may reveal a silent choroid in most patients because the lipofuscin in the RPE blocks the appearance of dye in the choroidal vessels (Fig. 6-26).

● Later in the disease, there may be fluorescein hyperfluorescence in the atrophic central macula.

● Early electroretinogram findings may be normal, but a subset of patients do have changes with prolonged dark adaptation. Multifocal electroretinography usually shows mild abnormalities.

Differential Diagnosis

● Fundus albipunctata

● Retinitis punctate albescens

● Cone dystrophy

● Batten's disease

● Hydroxychloroquine toxicity

● Autosomal dominant drusen

● Multifocal best

● Doyne's honeycomb

● Sorsby's dystrophy

● Malattia leventinese

● Bestrophinopathy

Diagnostic Evaluation

● Decreased vision in a child with classic dark choroid on angiography and sometimes yellow pisciform subretinal lesions are diagnostic.

● Visual field testing most commonly reveals a central scotoma, but paracentral and other variants may be seen.

● Electroretinogram findings may be helpful to rule out other causes of pediatric vision loss but are often normal in early Stargardt's disease.

● Genetic testing of the patient and other family members is often helpful.

Treatment

- Genetic counseling and low vision services are recommended. No other specific treatments have proven effective to date.
- Avoid vitamin A supplementation.

Prognosis

- Some variants of fundus flavimaculata are associated with better visual prognosis, but

Stargardt's disease is generally associated with moderate to poor central visual acuity.

REFERENCES

Goodwin P. Hereditary retinal disease. *Curr Opin Ophthalmol.* 2008;19:255–262.

Oh KT, Weleber RG, Stone EM, et al. Electroretinographic findings in patients with Stargardt disease and fundus flavimaculatus. *Retina.* 2004;24(6):920–928.

Westerfeld C, Mukai S. Stargardt's disease and the ABCR gene. *Semin Ophthalmol.* 2008;23(1):59–65.

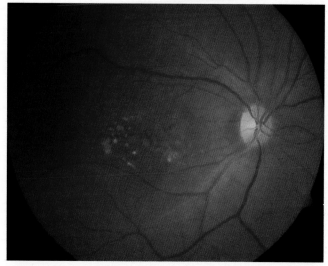

FIGURE 6-25. Stargardt's disease or fundus flavimaculata. Fundus photographs with macular yellow subretinal flecks.

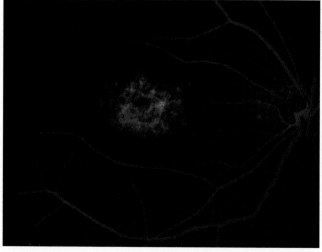

FIGURE 6-26. Fluorescein angiogram revealing dark or silent choroid because lipofuscin in the retinal pigment epithelium blocks choroidal vessel.

Eyelid Anomalies

Kammi B. Gunton ■

ANKYLOBLEPHARON

Etiology

- Ectodermal dysplasia, otherwise unknown

- In ankyloblepharon–ectodermal dysplasia–clefting (AEC) patients, a defect in the *TP63* gene, an epidermis intercellular junction regulator protein, is deficient. AEC is inherited in autosomal dominant fashion.

Symptoms

- Poor eyelid opening

Signs

- Partial or complete fusion of eyelid margins along portion of their length by webs of skin (Fig. 7-1)

- Shortened palpebral fissure

- Internal ankyloblepharon has fusion along inner canthus

- External ankyloblepharon has fusion of margin along outer canthus and is more common

- In ankyloblepharon filiforme adnatum variant, fine strands of skin connect margins.

- Associated with cleft lip, cleft palate, and ectodermal defects called AEC. Patients have ankyloblepharon filiforme adnatum; ectodermal defects such as sparse wiry hair, skin erosions, pigmentary changes, nail dystrophy, or dental abnormalities; and cleft lip or palate.

Differential Diagnosis

- Cryptophthalmos, failure of differentiation of eyelid structures; the cornea is attached to eyelid skin

- Congenital coloboma, defect within the eyelid, small notch or entire eyelid absent

- Epiblepharon, with extra fold of orbicularis, in the lower eyelid, turning eyelashes inward; no attachment between eyelids

Diagnostic Evaluation

- External examination of the eyelids reveals strands or a web of skin attaching the eyelid margin.

- Underlying cornea and eye structures are intact and unaffected.

- In AEC, molecular genetic testing for *TP63* mutations

Treatment

- Spontaneous resolution with ankyloblepharon filiforme adnatum is possible.

- Otherwise, hemostat to connective tissue followed by excision or skin strands or webs. Edges of conjunctiva and eyelid margin are apposed with sutures to prevent readhesion of skin.

Prognosis

- Excellent prognosis with treatment

- Prevent readhesion of skin

REFERENCES

Lopardo T, Loiacono N, Marinari B, et al. Claudin-1 is a p63 target gene with a crucial role in epithelial development. *PLoS One.* 2008;3(7):e2715.

Sumita S, Mridula M, Rainath, et al. What's your diagnosis? Diagnosis of ankyloblepharon filiforme adnatum. *J Pediatr Ophthalmol Strabismus.* 2010;47:139, 177.

Sutton VR, Bree AF, van Bokhoven H. Ankyloblepharon-ectodermal defects-cleft lip/palate syndrome. In Pagon RA, Bird TC, Dolan CR, et al, eds. *GeneReviews.* Seattle: University of Washington; 2008.

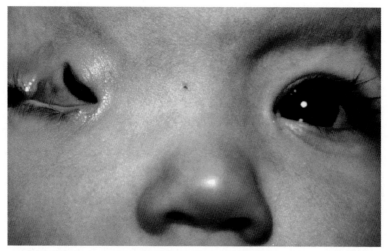

FIGURE 7-1. Ankyloblepharon with coloboma, right eyelid. (Courtesy of Robert Penne, MD, Department of Oculoplastics, Wills Eye Hospital, Philadelphia.)

BLEPHAROPHIMOSIS SYNDROME

Etiology

- Autosomal dominant inheritance
- Associated with *FOXL2* mutations

Symptoms

- Present congenitally
- Severe ptosis may cause ametropic amblyopia with blurred vision.

Signs

- Shortened palpebral length with three associated major signs: telecanthus (widened intercanthal distance), epicanthus inversus, and severe ptosis (Fig. 7-2)
- Additional signs include lower eyelid entropion, a poorly developed nasal bridge, hypoplasia of superior orbital rim, low-set ears, a short philtrum, lacrimal duct anomalies, refractive errors, and hypertelorism. Type I blepharophimosis syndrome (BPES) is associated with ovarian dysfunction, leading to premature ovarian failure.
- Type II BPES without ovarian dysfunction and premature ovarian failure

Differential Diagnosis

- Congenital ptosis; would occur with absence of other features
- Epicanthus, isolated finding

Diagnostic Evaluation

- Based on the presence of four classic signs: blepharophimosis, ptosis, epicanthus inversus, and telecanthus
- Testing for *FOXL2* may help in the diagnosis.
- Evaluation for ovarian dysfunction is needed.

Treatment

- Staged surgical treatment of signs, including multiple Z-, Y-, or V-plasties and intranasal wiring of medial canthus tendons to correct telecanthus at age 3 to 5 years followed 1 year later by bilateral frontal sling or levator resection as indicated for ptosis. With bilateral ametropic amblyopia, ptosis repair may need to be expedited.
- Simultaneous medial canthoplasty and blepharoptosis correction in select patients

Prognosis

- With surgical correction, improved cosmesis
- Visual prognosis is guarded because of amblyopia development. The timing of surgical correction is critical to prevent amblyopia.
- Ovarian dysfunction is treated with hormone replacement therapy, and reproductive issues may be addressed with reproduce technologies, including embryo or egg donation.

REFERENCES

Beysen D, DePaepe A, DeBaere E. FOXL2 mutations and genomic rearrangements in BPES. *Hum Mutat.* 2009;30:158–169.

DeBaere E. Blepharophimosis, ptosis, and epicanthus inversus. In: Pagon RA, Bird TC, Dolan CR, Stephens K, eds. *GeneReviews.* Seattle: University of Washington; 2009.

Huang WQ, Qiao Q, Zhao R, et al. Surgical strategy for congenital blepharophimosis syndrome. *Chin Med J.* 2007;120:1413–1415.

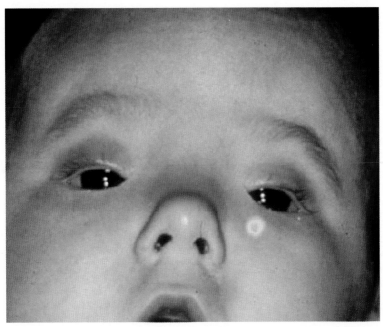

FIGURE 7-2. Child with blepharophimosis syndrome. Note blepharophimosis with telecanthus (widened intercanthal distance) epicanthus inversus, and severe ptosis. (Courtesy of Robert Penne, MD, Department of Oculoplastics, Wills Eye Hospital, Philadelphia.)

CONGENITAL ECTROPION

Etiology

- Congenital; classified as primary or secondary

- Primary resulting from absence or atrophy of tarsal plate

- Secondary resulting from paralytic, cicatricial, or mechanical causes in childhood with vertical shortage of anterior lamella such as congenital malformations with skin retraction, trauma, burns, ichthyosis (cicatricial), inflammatory conditions from medications, birth trauma, allergies with orbicularis spasm, or tumors (mechanical)

- May occur in association with BPES, euryblepharon, microphthalmos, orbital cysts, and Down's syndrome

Symptoms

- Chronic epiphora, conjunctival injection, foreign body sensation, photophobia, reduced vision

Signs

- Eversion of eyelid margin; the lower eyelid is more commonly involved because of a vertical deficiency of skin (Fig. 7-3)

- Exposure keratitis and conjunctivitis

Differential Diagnosis

- Congenital tarsal kink: upper eyelid bent back with 180-degree fold of the upper tarsal plate

- Congenital entropion: distal portion of lower tarsal plate bent inward

- Euryblepharon: downward displacement of temporal portion of lower eyelid caused by enlargement of the lateral aperture

Diagnostic Evaluation

- Based on external examination with eversion of the eyelid

Treatment

- Mild cases require lubrication with artificial tears or ointments.

- With corneal exposure, surgical repair is required with lateral tarsorrhaphy or lateral canthoplasty to eliminate horizontal eyelid laxity to reposition the eyelid to the globe.

- In severe cases, a full-thickness skin graft is required.

- In tarsus agenesis, auricular cartilage may be used in the graft.

Prognosis

- With surgical correction, and skin graft in cases of vertical deficiency of skin, good prognosis

- Must prevent permanent corneal scarring from exposure keratitis, with resulting amblyopia

REFERENCES

Bedran EG, Pereira MV, Bernandes TF. Ectropion. *Semin Ophthalmol.* 2010;25:59–65.

Hintschich C. Correction of entropion and ectropion. *Dev Ophthalmol.* 2008;41:85–102.

Piskiniene R. Eyelid malposition: lower lid entropion and ectropion. *Medicina (Kaunas).* 2006;42:881–884.

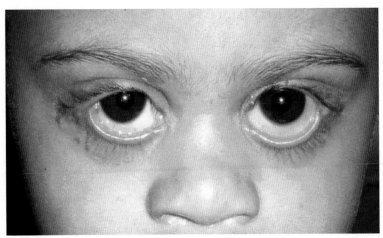

FIGURE 7-3. Ectropion. Note eversion of lower eyelids. (Courtesy of Jacqueline Carrasco, MD, Department of Oculoplastics, Wills Eye Hospital, Philadelphia.)

CONGENITAL ENTROPION

Etiology

- Rare as isolated defect (0.02%)
- Results from a lack of support to the posterior border of the eyelid, such as absence or kinking of the tarsal plate
- May have disinsertion or dysgenesis of the refractor layer of the eyelid
- Hereditary
- Equal sex distribution
- More common in Asians
- Often associated with epiblepharon, epicanthus, microphthalmos, and enophthalmos

Symptoms

- Epiphora, eyelid rubbing, photophobia
- Foreign body sensation, eye pain, conjunctival injection reduced vision

Signs

- Inward turning of eyelid
- Lower eyelid more commonly affected
- No skin fold in eyelid (**Fig. 7-4**)
- Corneal abrasion or keratitis from eyelash abrasions

Differential Diagnosis

- Epicanthus
- Epiblepharon

Diagnostic Evaluation

- External examination reveals inward turning of the eyelid margin.

- Evaluation for presence of the tarsal plate

Treatment

- Often spontaneous resolution as growth of facial bones corrects epiblepharon
- In the presence of corneal pathology with epiblepharon, surgical treatment to excise horizontal strip of orbicularis 3 mm from the eyelid border is required.
- Alternatively, capsulopalpebral muscle shortening or tightening of retractors of lower eyelid stops the preseptal orbicularis from riding over the pretarsal portion.
- Other surgical procedures include everting (Quickert) sutures; marginal rotation (Weis procedure); and in congenital tarsal kinking, horizontal tarsotomy with marginal rotation.

Prognosis

- If corneal scarring is prevented, good prognosis
- Risk for amblyopia and refractive error

REFERENCES

Katowitz WR, Katowitz JA. Congenital and developmental eyelid abnormalities. *Plast Reconstr Surg.* 2009; 124(suppl):93e–105e.

Naik MN, Honavar SG, Bhaduri A, et al. Congenital horizontal tarsal kink: a single-center experience with 6 cases. *Ophthalmology.* 2007;114:1564–1568.

Pereira MG, Rodrigues MA, Rodrigues SA. Eyelid entropion. *Semin Ophthalmol.* 2010;25:52–58.

Yang SW, Choi WC, Kim SY. Refractive changes of congenital entropion and epiblepharon on surgical correction. *Korean J Ophthalmol.* 2001;15:32–37.

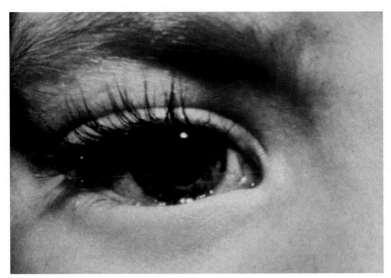

FIGURE 7-4. Congenital entropion. Inversion of the lower eyelid. (From Levin AV, Wilson TW, Pashby R, et al. Lids and adnexa. In: Levin AV, Wilson T, eds. *The Hospital for Sick Children's Atlas of Pediatric Ophthalmology.* Philadelphia: Lippincott Williams & Wilkins; 2007:31–39.)

CONGENITAL PTOSIS

Etiology

- Unknown
- Most histology studies support dysgenesis of levator palpebrae superioris muscle rather than dystrophy of muscle
- Equal sex distribution
- Unilateral and most commonly isolated finding

Symptoms

- Asymmetry of eyelid position, asymmetry of eyes, blurred vision

Signs

- Vertical shortening of the palpebral fissure caused by upper eyelid droop (Fig. 7-5)
- Normal upper eyelid position is 1 to 2 mm below the superior limbus.

Differential Diagnosis

- Marcus-Gunn jaw wink
- Third nerve palsy
- Horner's syndrome
- Myasthenia gravis

Diagnostic Evaluation

- Evaluation of eyelid position, margin–corneal reflex distance, levator excursion, presence of eyelid crease
- Evaluate for enophthalmos and extra ocular muscle functions, especially superior rectus and synergistic eye movements as well as pupillary responses

Treatment

- Multiple surgical treatments available depending on the degree of levator function and amount of droop, including frontalis sling; levator resection; Whitnall sling; and in limited cases with mild ptosis, Mullerectomy

Prognosis

- Evaluation for anisometropic amblyopia
- Concern for corneal exposure into adulthood, especially in the absence of Bell's phenomenon
- Recurrence of ptosis with facial growth, laxity in sutures for frontal sling

REFERENCES

Baldwin HC, Manners RM. Congenital blepharoptosis: a literature review of the histology of levator palpebrae superioris muscle. *Ophthalmol Plast Reconstr Surg.* 2002;18:301–307.

McMullan TF, Robinson DO, Tyers AG. Towards an understanding of congenital ptosis. *Orbit.* 2006; 25: 179–184.

Oral Y, Ozqur OR, Akcay L, et al. Congenital ptosis and amblyopia. *J Pediatr Ophthalmol Strabismus.* 2010; 47:101–104.

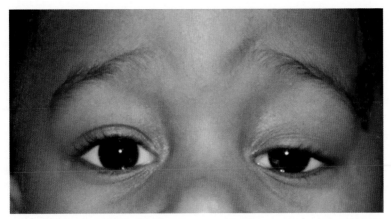

FIGURE 7-5. Congenital ptosis of the left eye.

EYELID COLOBOMAS

Etiology

- Localized failure of fusion of embryonic eyelid folds, failure of adhesion of eyelid folds, or premature breaking of adhesion, resulting in a lag of growth
- Trauma from amniotic bands
- Associated with craniofacial dysostosis, especially with lower, temporal eyelid involvement; also with limbal dermoids (Goldenhar's syndrome), conjunctiva chondroma, symblepharon, iris and fundus coloboma, eyebrow coloboma, and cleft palate
- No inheritance pattern for upper eyelid colobomas; loose dominant hereditary pattern for lower eyelid colobomas

Symptoms

- Epiphora with corneal, conjunctival exposure

Signs

- Defect in eyelid margin; varies from small defect to absence of length of eyelid (Fig. 7-6)
- May involve one or all four eyelids but most common in nasal portion of upper eyelid
- Edges of defect rounded and covered with conjunctiva

- Corneal epithelial erosion and ulceration with large colobomas

Differential Diagnosis

- Euryblepharon
- Congenital ectropion
- Tarsal kinking

Diagnostic Evaluation

- External examination with complete absence of portion of eyelid margin, including eyelashes

Treatment

- Up to one-third eyelid margin repaired with direct closure; lateral cantholysis can provide horizontal relaxation required for closure
- Eyelid sharing procedures such as Cutler-Beard and Hughes in children occlude visual axis, albeit temporarily, and may result in amblyopia

Prognosis

- Good cosmesis with surgical closure
- Prevent corneal scarring to prevent amblyopia.

REFERENCES

Ankola PA, Abdel-Azim H. Congenital bilateral upper eyelid coloboma. *J Perinatol.* 2003;23:166–167.
Betharia SM, Kumar S. Congenital colobomas of the eyelids. *Indian J Ophthalmol.* 1988;36:29–31.

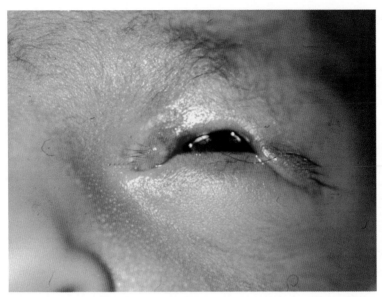

FIGURE 7-6. Upper eyelid coloboma. (Courtesy of Robert Penne, MD, Department of Oculoplastics, Wills Eye Hospital, Philadelphia.)

EPIBLEPHARON

Etiology

- Overriding pretarsal orbicularis with horizontal skin layer pushing the cilia vertically

- Possible etiologies for redundant skin include a weak attachment of the pretarsal orbicularis to the tarsus, hypertrophy of the orbicularis oculi, or failure of septae in the subcutaneous plane of the pretarsal orbicularis and overlying skin, resulting in poor adhesion between the lower eyelid retractors and skin or orbicularis.

- More common in Asians and involving lower eyelid and bilateral

- Associated with other eyelid conditions, including lower eyelid retraction

Symptoms

- Possibly none or vertical orientation of eyelashes

- Severe cases, foreign body sensation, epiphora, conjunctival injection, photophobia, eyelid rubbing

Signs

- Presence of excess horizontal skin along the upper or lower eyelid margin that forces cilia into a vertical position, often against ocular surface with blink (Fig. 7-7)

- Tarsus in a normal position relative to the globe

Differential Diagnosis

- Entropion: eyelid turned inward relative toward the globe

Diagnostic Evaluation

- External examination with eyelid margin in normal position relative to the globe; excess horizontal skin fold pushing cilia toward the globe into a vertical position

- Evaluation of the cornea for staining

Treatment

- In the absence of corneal pathology, no treatment is indicated. Subsequently, facial growth frequently eliminates corneal and eyelash touch.

- Appropriate lubrication with ointments to protect corneal surface before surgical correction when corneal keratitis is detected

- If required, horizontal skin 3 mm from the eyelid margin is excised with the underlying orbicularis; reapproximation is done of the skin edges, pulling the cilia away from the ocular surface.

- Alternatively, the above procedure is combined with thermal cautery to the orbital septum, allowing adhesion of the septum to the preseptal orbicularis and preventing overriding of muscle and sutures in the inferior tarsus and upper skin flap to further rotate cilia from ocular surface.

- Small injection of hyaluronic acid gel above the overriding pretarsal orbicularis was recently reported to relieve cilial–corneal touch for up to 6 months.

Prognosis

- Spontaneous resolution in the majority of cases with facial growth

- Primary excision of pretarsal orbicularis is highly effective with only 5% recurrence rate at 6 months. Patients with Down's syndrome may have a slightly higher recurrence rate.

REFERENCES

Kakizaki H, Leibovitch I, Takahashi Y, et al. Eyelash inversion in epiblepharon: is it caused by redundant skin? *Clin Ophthalmol.* 2009;3:247–250.

Lee KM, Choung HK, Kim NJ, et al. Prognosis of upper eyelid epiblepharon repair in Down syndrome. *Am J Ophthalmol.* 2010;150:476–480.e1.

Lee H, Park M, Lee TE, et al. Surgical correction of epiblepharon using thermal cauterization of the orbital septum and lash-rotating sutures. *J Craniofac Surg.* 2010; 21:1069–1071.

Naik MN, Ali MJ, Das S, et al. Nonsurgical management of epiblepharon using hyaluronic acid gel. *Ophthalmol Plast Reconstr Surg.* 2010;26:215–217.

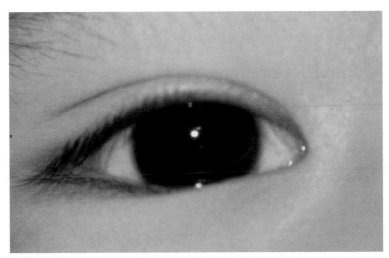

FIGURE 7-7. Epiblepharon. Note the excess horizontal skin in the lower eyelid margin pushing cilia into a vertical position. (Courtesy of Alex Levin, MD, Department of Pediatric Ophthalmology, Wills Eye Hospital, Philadelphia.)

EPICANTHUS

Etiology

- Usually bilateral; can be isolated or associated with ptosis or BPES, especially epicanthus inversus

- More common in Asians

- When associated with BPES, the *FOXL2* gene is implicated.

- Histologic studies show possible congenital dysplasia of the medial canthal tendon with disorganized collagen in BPES contributing to epicanthus.

Symptoms

- None

Signs

- Semilunar fold of skin extending from upper eyelid medially to the margin of the lower eyelid

- Four types:

  - Tarsalis: fold of skin most prominent in upper eyelid; most common (Fig. 7-8)

  - Inversus: skin fold arises from below the canthus; prominent in lower eyelid

  - Palpebralis: fold equally distributed between the upper and lower eyelids

  - Supraciliaris: skin fold originates above the canthus from the eyebrow region

Differential Diagnosis

- BPES

Diagnostic Evaluation

- External examination of eyelids with notation of skin fold origination site and prominent eyelid involvement

Treatment

- Most often none required; facial growth diminishes appearance

- If desired after facial maturity, reconstruction of eyelid with Z-plasty or Y-V-plasty of skin fold

Prognosis

- Good cosmesis with surgical correction when desired

REFERENCES

Katowitz WR, Katowitz JA. Congenital and developmental eyelid abnormalities. *Plast Reconstr Surg.* 2009; 124(suppl):93e–105e.

Ruban JM, Baggio E. Surgical treatment of congenital eyelid malpositions in children. *J Fr Ophthalmol.* 2004; 27:304–326.

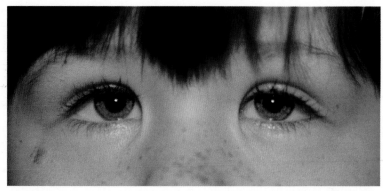

FIGURE 7-8. Epicanthus, tarsalis. (Courtesy of Alex Levin, MD, Department of Pediatric Ophthalmology, Wills Eye Hospital, Philadelphia.)

CAPILLARY HEMANGIOMAS

Etiology

- Most common vascular orbital tumor of childhood
- Unencapsulated lesion with lobules of endothelial cells lining blood–filled spaces with intervening fibrous septa
- More common in females, whites, and premature births
- Present at birth to several months of life; rapid growth for 3 to 6 months in the proliferative phase followed by the involutional phase with fibrofatty deposition around endothelial cells with fibrosis and involution of the lesion
- During the proliferative phase, basic fibroblast growth factor (bFGF), and vascular endothelial growth factor (VEGF) play a role.

Symptoms

- Blurred vision, ptosis

Signs

- Classic superficial strawberry nevus mass lesion in the orbit (Fig. 7-9)
- Subcutaneous, blue- to purple-colored mass lesion in the orbit
- Proptosis without skin discoloration from deep orbital hemangiomas
- Reduced vision; anisometropic astigmatism

Differential Diagnosis

- Lymphangioma: no overlying strawberry nevus, episodic hemorrhages around orbit
- Rhabdomyosarcoma: rapid growth with proptosis
- Orbital dermoid: classic superotemporal location, slow growth

Diagnostic Evaluation

- External examination and imaging study as needed to determine the extent of the hemangioma

Treatment

- In the presence of anisometropic astigmatism and amblyopia, options for treatment include oral steroids, intralesional steroids, argon laser, surgical excision, and oral and perhaps topical propranolol.
- Propranolol titrated up to 2 mg/kg/day divided three times a day. A response in size is seen in 24 hours. Oral treatment may be needed for up to 12 months. Because of the possible side effects of bradycardia, hypotension, and hypoglycemia, monitoring is required. Residual scarring may occur with treatment. Topical β-blocker therapy is also under investigation.
- Propranolol causes rapid vasoconstriction and may reduce expression of VEGF and bFGF or promote apoptosis of capillary endothelial cells to reduce the hemangioma.

Prognosis

- The involutional phase occurs over 5 to 7 years. Complete resolution occurs in 75% to 90% of children by age 7 years.
- Amblyopia is difficult to treat and more common in upper eyelid lesions, nasal eyelid location, lesions larger than 1 cm, and diffuse orbital lesions.

REFERENCES

Guo S, Ni N. Topical treatment for capillary hemangioma of the eyelid using beta-blocker solution. *Arch Ophthalmol*. 2010;128:255–256.

Leaute-Labreze C, Dumas de la Roque E, Hubiche T, et al. Propranolol for severe hemangiomas of infancy. *N Engl J Med*. 2008; 358:2649–2651.

Schwartz SR, Blei F, Ceisler E, et al. Risk Factors for amblyopia in children with capillary hemangiomas of the eyelids and orbit. *J AAPOS*. 2006;10:262–268.

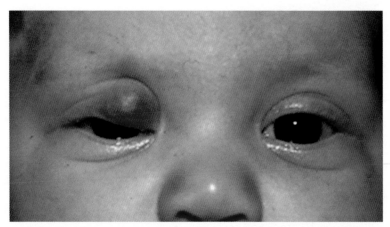

FIGURE 7-9. Right upper eyelid capillary hemangioma. (Courtesy of Judith Lavrich, MD, Department of Pediatric Ophthalmology, Wills Eye Hospital, Philadelphia.)

Lacrimal Anomalies

Leonard B. Nelson and Harold P. Koller ■

CONGENITAL MUCOCELE

- When an obstruction at the upper and lower portions of the lacrimal system occurs, fluid accumulates and causes a distention of the lacrimal sac at birth, termed a *mucocele.*

Etiology

- Sporadic
- Concomitant blockage at the valve of Rosenmüller and in the nasolacrimal duct leads to the formation of lacrimal sac mucoceles.

Symptoms

- Tearing
- Difficulty breathing
- Difficulty with breastfeeding on the mother's breast ipsilateral to the mucocele

Signs

- Blue-gray swelling inferior to the medial canthal tendon at birth (Fig. 8-1).
- Secondary infection (erythema of the tissues overlying the lacrimal sac) may occur.

- Mucocele may extend intranasally as a submucocele mass along the nasal floor beneath the inferior turbinate.

Differential Diagnosis

- Hemangioma
- Dermoid
- Encephalocele
- Nasal glioma

Treatment

- Conservative management includes gentle massage and warm compresses.
- Dacryocystitis can develop within a few days or weeks and requires systemic antibiotics.
- Ultimately, if the mucocele cannot be decompressed with massage, within several days, prompt probing has been recommended. Rarely, serious complications of central nervous system infections have been reported; therefore, some have recommended early probing.

Prognosis

- The resolution rate with conservative management is approximately 76%.

- If probing is necessary, resolution can be accomplished.

REFERENCES

Harris GJ, DiClementi D. Congenital dacryocystocele. *Arch Ophthalmol.* 1982;100:1763–1765.

Schnall BM, Christain CJ. Conservative treatment of congenial dacryocele. *J Pediatr Ophthal Strabismus.* 1996;33:219–222.

Wong RK, VanderVeen DK. Presentation and management of congenital dacryocystocele. *Pediatrics.* 2008;122: 1108–1112.

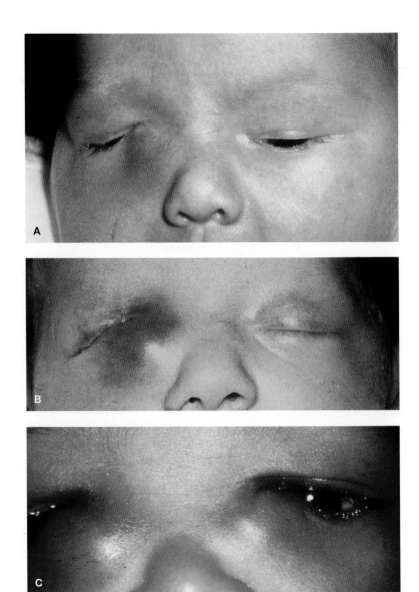

FIGURE 8-1. A. Mucocele of the nasolacrimal system showing swelling and mild erythema. **B.** Mucocele showing more significant swelling and erythema. **C.** Bilateral mucoceles.

CONGENITAL NASOLACRIMAL DUCT OBSTRUCTION

- Congenital nasolacrimal duct obstruction (NLDO) is the most common abnormality of infants' lacrimal apparatus, occurring in 2% to 6% of infants.

Etiology

- Sporadic
- An imperforate membrane at the distal level of the nasolacrimal duct is the usual cause of occlusion

Symptoms

- Usually presents within the first weeks of life with persistent epiphora and intermittent mucopurulent discharge

Signs

- Typically, the tears spill over the lower eyelid, and there is a "wet look" in the involved eye(s) (Fig. 8-2).
- Eyelashes may be matted together from mucus discharge.
- Conjunctiva usually appears white and uninflamed.

Diagnostic Evaluation

- Clinical history, symptoms, and signs are usually enough to establish diagnosis. Rarely, ethmoiditis can contribute to a resistant mucopurulent discharge and may need to be investigated.
- Can perform fluorescein dye disappearance test

Treatment

- Although controversy continues to exist, most studies have shown spontaneous remittance in 80% to 90% of affected infants by 12 months of age.
- Massage, eyelid hygiene, and occasional antibiotic treatment
- If symptoms are still present by 13 months of age, probing is required.
- If repeated probing is necessary and does not eliminate symptoms, the patient may require intubation with silicone tubing or balloon catheter.

Prognosis

- Most congenital NLDOs resolve spontaneously before age 1 and do not need probing.
- Most NLDOs that require probing are cured with that procedure and do not require an intubation or balloon catheter.

REFERENCES

Becker BB, Berry FD, Koller H. Balloon catheter dilation for treatment of congenital nasolacrimal duct obstruction. *Am J Ophthalmol.* 1996;121:304–309.

El-Mansoury J, Calhoun JH, Nelson LB, et al. Results of late probing for congenital nasolacrimal duct obstruction. *Ophthalmology.* 1986;93:1052–1054.

Nelson LB, Calhoun JH, Menduke H. Medical management of congenital nasolacrimal duct obstruction. *J Pediatric Ophthalmol Strabismus.* 1985;76:172–175.

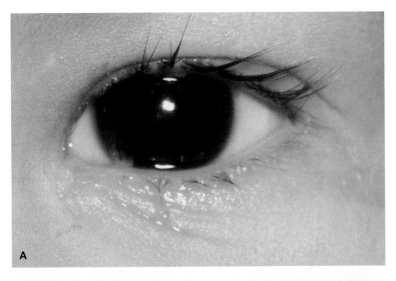

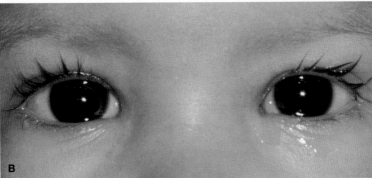

FIGURE 8-2. **A.** Nasolacrimal duct obstruction showing the "wet look," with matting of the lashes. **B.** Bilateral nasolacrimal duct obstruction, tearing, and matting of the lashes. Notice that the conjunctiva is clear.

Strabismus Disorders

Scott E. Olitsky and Leonard B. Nelson ■

PSEUDOESOTROPIA

Epidemiology and Etiology

- Pseudoesotropia is one of the most common reasons an ophthalmologist is asked to evaluate an infant. In some series, up to half of children with suspected strabismus were found to have pseudoesotropia.

- Pseudoesotropia is characterized by the false appearance of strabismus when the visual axes are actually aligned (Fig. 9-1).

History

- Pseudoesotropia is usually caused by a flat, broad nasal bridge; prominent epicanthal folds; or a narrow interpupillary distance. An observer may perceive less white sclera nasally than would be expected, and the impression is that the eye is turned in toward the nose, especially when the child looks to either side.

Differential Diagnosis

- Small-angle strabismus
- Intermittent strabismus

Diagnostic Evaluation

- Pseudoesotropia can be differentiated from true strabismus when the corneal light reflex is seen to be centered in both eyes or when the cover–uncover test shows no refixation movement.

- Tightening the epicanthal folds by pinching the bridge of the nose can also be effective in demonstrating that the "crossing" is not real.

- A complete evaluation should be performed, including cycloplegic refraction, to rule out excessive hyperopia that could be causing intermittent esotropia.

Treatment

- No treatment is needed. Parents can be reassured that most children will outgrow the appearance of crossing.

Prognosis

- As the child grows, the bridge of the nose becomes more prominent and displaces the epicanthal folds, and the medial sclera becomes proportional to the amount visible on the lateral aspect of the eye. Parents should be cautioned that children with pseudoesotropia, like any child, can develop true strabismus later in life. Therefore, if a change in appearance occurs, a repeat evaluation may be warranted.

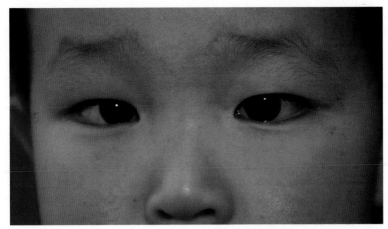

FIGURE 9-1. Pseudoesotropia caused by a wide nasal bridge and epicanthal folds. Note that the child is looking slightly to the left which also accentuates the fale appearance that there is less sclera in the right eye.

CONGENITAL (INFANTILE) ESOTROPIA

Epidemiology and Etiology

• The cause of congenital esotropia is unknown. Theories include both a primary defect in sensory development of the brain that leads to the abnormal alignment as well as a primary "motor" theory in which the ocular misalignment is the primary abnormality, which then leads to a secondary disruption of binocular vision. It is likely that both causes exist and may also be equally responsible for the development of the disorder in many children.

The incidence of congenital esotropia is approximately 1 in 1000 children.

Signs and Symptoms

• Few children who are eventually diagnosed with this disorder are actually born with an esotropia. Although parents often give a history of their child's eyes crossing since birth, the crossing is rarely seen in the newborn nursery and is generally not observed during the first few weeks of life.

• The diagnosis is generally made when an infant presents before 6 months of age with a large ($\geq$30 prism diopter), constant esotropia, full abduction, a normal level of hyperopia, and no underlying ophthalmic disorder that could lead to vision loss and a secondary strabismus (Fig. 9-2). Children with congenital esotropia often appear to exhibit an apparent abduction deficit. This pseudoparesis is usually secondary to the presence of cross-fixation. If the child has equal vision, he or she will have no need to abduct either eye. The child will use the adducted, or crossed, eye to look to the opposite field of gaze. In this case, he or she will show a bilateral pseudoparesis of abduction. If amblyopia is present, only the better-seeing eye will cross fixate, making the amblyopic eye appear to have an abduction weakness. To differentiate between a true abducens paralysis and a pseudoparalysis, a doll's head maneuver can be used or abduction can be examined after the infant has worn a patch over one eye for a period of time.

Differential Diagnosis

• Pseudoesotropia
• Duane's retraction syndrome
• Mobius syndrome
• Congenital sixth nerve palsy
• Early-onset accommodative esotropia
• Sensory esotropia
• Esotropia in the neurologically impaired

Diagnostic Evaluation

• All children with suspected congenital esotropia should under a complete examination, including a dilated funduscopic evaluation and cycloplegic refraction to rule out possible early onset accommodative esotropia or a secondary strabismus (Fig. 9-3).

• Amblyopia can be diagnosed by looking for a fixation preference.

• If an accommodative component to the crossing is considered to be a possibility, the child should be given the full cycloplegic refraction and reevaluated to look for any effect on the crossing.

Treatment

• The treatment for congenital esotropia consists of strabismus surgery. Surgery is performed after any associated amblyopia, if present, is treated. It is important to treat amblyopia before surgery. It is much easier to follow the progress of amblyopia in a preverbal child while his or her eyes are crossed. In addition, parental compliance with amblyopia treatment tends to be much lower after the eyes are straightened and appear "normal."

- The primary goal of treatment in congenital esotropia is to eliminate or reduce the deviation as much as possible. Ideally, this results in normal visual acuity in each eye, straight-looking eyes, and the development of binocular vision.

Prognosis

- Children with congenital esotropia do not develop normal (bifoveal) binocular vision. Successful treatment provides the opportunity to develop some degree of binocular vision (monofixation syndrome), which allows the development of motor fusion, which helps to keep their eyes aligned.

- Even with successful initial treatment, many children with a history of congenital esotropia may redevelop strabismus or amblyopia and therefore need to be monitored closely during the visually immature period of life.

- Recurrent horizontal strabismus is common as are vertical deviations. These may develop months or years after the initial surgery has been performed. The two most common forms of vertical deviations to develop are inferior oblique muscle overaction (IOOA) and dissociated vertical deviation (DVD).

REFERENCES

Archer SM, Sondhi N, Helveston EM. Strabismus in infancy. *Ophthalmology.* 1989;96:133.

Arthur BW, Smith JT, Scott WE. Long-term stability of alignment in the monofixation syndrome. *J Pediatr Ophthalmol Strabismus.* 1989;26:224.

Birch E, Stager D, Wright K, et al. The natural history of infantile esotropia during the first six months of life. *J AAPOS.* 1998;2:325–328.

Birch EE, Stager DR, Everett ME. Random dot stereoacuity following surgical correction of infantile esotropia. *J Pediatr Ophthalmol Strabismus.* 1995;32:231.

Hiles DA, Watson A, Biglan AW. Characteristics of infantile esotropia following early bimedial rectus recession. *Arch Ophthalmol.* 1980;98:697.

Ing M, Costenbader FD, Parks MM, et al. Early surgery for congenital esotropia. *Am J Ophthalmol.* 1966;62:1419.

Parks MM. The monofixation syndrome. *Trans Am Ophthalmol Soc.* 1969;67:609.

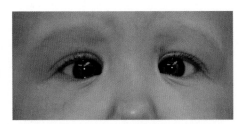

FIGURE 9-2. Congenital (infantile) esotropia. (From Nelson LB, Olitsky SE. *A Color Handbook of Pediatric Clinical Ophthalmology.* London: Manson Publishing, 2011.)

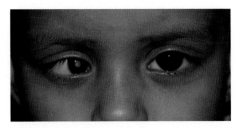

FIGURE 9-3. Sensory esotropia secondary to a congenital cataract in the right eye.

INFERIOR OBLIQUE OVERACTION

Epidemiology and Etiology

• Inferior oblique overaction occurs in a primary and secondary form. Most patients with primary IOOA have history of congenital esotropia, but it may occur in association with other forms of strabismus as well. Up to 80% of patients with a history of congenital esotropia may develop IOOA. Secondary IOOA occurs in patients with superior oblique palsy.

Signs and Symptoms

• IOOA results in elevation of the involved eye as it moves nasally (**Fig. 9-4**).

Differential Diagnosis

• DVD

• Duane's syndrome with upshoot

Diagnostic Evaluation

• The amount of overaction is evaluated in the field of action of the inferior oblique muscle in question. IOOA can be classified as grades I to IV. Grade I represents 1 mm of higher elevation of the adducting eye in gaze up and to the side. Grade IV indicates 4 mm of higher elevation. These differences in elevation between the two eyes are measured from the 6 o'clock position on each limbus. A measurement of the degree of adduction that is required to elicit the overaction is also helpful when considering treatment.

Treatment

• IOOA can be treated surgically. The thresholds for surgery for IOOA are different, depending on whether weakening the inferior oblique is the only surgery being contemplated or whether weakening the inferior oblique in conjunction with horizontal strabismus surgery is being considered. If the inferior obliques alone are weakened, there should be a significant overaction present to justify surgery. If horizontal surgery is being performed, smaller grades of inferior oblique overaction may be corrected at the same time. Inferior oblique recession, myotomy, myectomy or denervation and extirpation can be performed to weaken the action of the inferior oblique.

• Anterior transposition of the inferior oblique can also be performed to limit the elevation of the eye and may be the treatment of choice when both IOOA and DVD occur together.

Prognosis

• Surgery is generally successful at improving the overacting inferior oblique muscle. Care must be taken to not miss any fibers of the muscle at the time of surgery.

REFERENCE

Parks MM. A study of the weakening surgical procedure for eliminating overaction of the inferior oblique. *Am J Ophthalmol.* 1972;73:107.

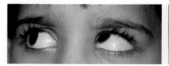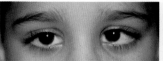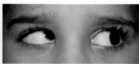

FIGURE 9-4. Inferior oblique overaction in both eyes. Note the elevation of each eye in adduction.

DISSOCIATED VERTICAL DEVIATION

Epidemiology and Etiology

● Most patients with DVD have history of congenital esotropia, but it may occur in association with other forms of strabismus as well.

● Up to 90% of patients with a history of congenital esotropia may develop DVD.

● DVD appears to be a time-related phenomenon and is not related to successful initial surgery or the development of binocular vision.

Signs and Symptoms

● DVD consists of a slow upward deviation of one or alternate eyes (Fig. 9-5). Excyclotorsion can often be demonstrated on upward drifting of the eye and incyclotorsion on downward motion.

● DVD may be latent, detected only when the involved eye is covered, or manifest, occurring intermittently or constantly. It can be differentiated from a true vertical deviation because no corresponding hypotropia occurs in the other eye on cover testing.

Differential Diagnosis

● Inferior oblique overaction

● Hypertropia

Diagnostic Evaluation

● DVD can be estimated by using the Hirschberg and Krimsky methods or the prism-cover test. A base-down prism is placed over the involved eye. The strength of the prism is adjusted until no movement occurs as the cover is shifted from the involved to the fixating eye. Because prism-cover measurement is difficult and may be inaccurate, DVD can also be estimated using a semiquantitative grading scale (1 to 4+).

Treatment

● If amblyopia exists, improvement in vision may improve fusional control and decrease how frequently the deviation is manifest.

● If DVD is entirely latent, detected on cover testing only, surgery is not indicated. If it is intermittent, surgery is determined by the size and frequency of the deviation as well as the patient's concern regarding it's appearance. Surgical treatment for DVD includes recession of the superior rectus and recession of the superior rectus combined with a posterior fixation suture and anterior transposition of the inferior oblique (preferred if IOOA coexists).

Prognosis

● It is often not possible to completely eliminate DVD. The goal of treatment is to reduce the magnitude of the deviation enough that it is not noticeable when it is manifest.

REFERENCES

Bacal DA, Nelson LB. Anterior transposition of the inferior oblique muscle for both dissociated vertical deviation and/or inferior oblique overaction: results of 94 procedures in 55 patients. *Binocular Vision Eye Muscle Surg.* 1992;7:219.

Mims JL, Wood RC. Bilateral anterior transposition of the inferior obliques. *Arch Ophthalmol.* 1989;107:41.

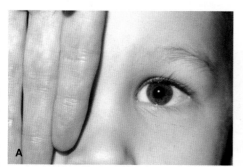 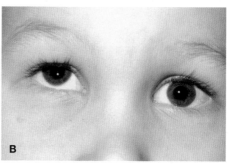

FIGURE 9-5. Dissociated vertical deviation. **A.** Right eye occluded. **B.** Dissociated vertical deviation manifest after occlusion. (Courtesy of Alex Levin, MD.)

REFRACTIVE ACCOMMODATIVE ESOTROPIA

Epidemiology and Etiology

- The mechanism of refractive accommodative esotropia involves three factors: uncorrected hyperopia, accommodative convergence, and insufficient fusional divergence. When an individual exerts a given amount of accommodation, a specific amount of convergence (accommodative convergence) is associated with it. An uncorrected hyperope must exert excessive accommodation to clear a blurred retinal image. This in turn stimulates excessive convergence. If the amplitude of fusional divergence is sufficient to correct the excess convergence, no esotropia will result. However, if the fusional divergence amplitudes are inadequate or motor fusion is altered by some sensory obstacle, an esotropia will result.

Signs and Symptoms

- Refractive accommodative esotropia usually occurs in a child between 2 and 3 years of age with a history of acquired intermittent or constant esotropia. Occasionally, children who are 1 year of age or younger present with accommodative esotropia.

- The refraction of patients with refractive accommodative esotropia averages +4.75 diopters. The angle of esodeviation is the same when measured at distance and near fixation and is usually moderate in magnitude, ranging between 20 and 40 prism diopters.

Amblyopia is common, especially when the esodeviation has become more nearly constant.

Differential Diagnosis

- Congenital esotropia
- Nonaccommodative esotropia
- Nonrefractive accommodative esotropia

Diagnostic Evaluation

- A complete examination should be performed, including a cycloplegic refraction.

Treatment

- The full hyperopic correction, determined by cycloplegic refraction, should be prescribed.

Prognosis

- Most children will maintain straight eyes while wearing their glasses (Fig. 9-6). Some children may show an increase in their hyperopia, which can lead to a recurrent crossing. A nonaccommodative esotropia may develop in a small percentage of children. Patients with relatively smaller levels of hyperopia may eventually outgrow their need for glasses as their hyperopic refractive error lessens with age.

REFERENCES

Coats DK, Avilla CW, Paysse EA, et al. Early-onset refractive accommodative esotropia. *J AAPOS*. 1998; 2:275–278.

Raab EL. Etiologic factors in accommodative esodeviation. *Trans Am Ophthalmol Soc*. 1982;80:657.

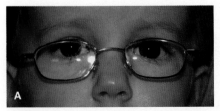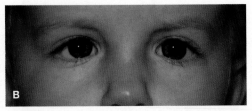

FIGURE 9-6. Refractive accommodative esotropia. **A.** With the appropriate hyperopic glasses the eyes are straight. **B.** Without glasses there is an esotropia of 25 prism diopters.

NONREFRACTIVE ACCOMMODATIVE ESOTROPIA

Epidemiology and Etiology

- Children with nonrefractive accommodative esotropia usually present between 2 and 3 years of age with an esodeviation that is greater at near than at distance fixation. The refractive error in this condition may be hyperopic or myopic, although the average refraction is +2.25 diopters.

- In nonrefractive accommodative esotropia, there is a high accommodative convergence to accommodation (AC:A) ratio: The effort to accommodate elicits an abnormally high accommodative convergence response.

Signs and Symptoms

- Some parents notice the crossing that only takes place at near fixation.

- There are a number of ways of measuring the AC:A ratio. Most clinicians prefer to assess the ratio using the distance–near comparison. The AC:A relationship is derived by simply comparing the distance and near deviation. If the near measurement in a patient with esotropia is greater than 10 prism diopters, the AC:A ratio is considered to be abnormally high.

Differential Diagnosis

- Refractive accommodative esotropia

Diagnostic Evaluation

- A complete examination, including a measurement of the esotropia at both distance and near fixation as well as a cycloplegic refraction, should be performed.

Treatment

- Treatment often uses the use of bifocal lenses to eliminate the accommodative effort required for near work. The bifocal is usually prescribed as an executive type lens that bisects the pupil.

- Other treatment options include miotics and strabismus surgery. Some patients may be followed because those with good alignment at distance usually develop normal vision.

Prognosis

- Many patients show a normalization of their AC:A ratio over time.

- Some patients decompensate and develop a nonaccommodative component that may require surgery. The risk of decompensation appears to be related to the magnitude of the distance–near disparity of the crossing.

REFERENCES

Kushner BJ. Fifteen-year outcome of surgery for the near angle in patients with accommodative esotropia and a high accommodative convergence to accommodation ratio. *Arch Ophthalmol.* 2001;119:1150–1153.

Ludwig IH, Parks MM, Getson PR. Long-term results of bifocal therapy for accommodative esotropia. *J Pediatr Ophthalmol Strabismus.* 1989;26:264.

O'Hara MA, Calhoun JH. Surgical correction of excess esotropia at near. *J Pediatr Ophthalmol Strabismus.* 1990;27:120.

Pratt-Johnson JA, Tillson G. The management of esotropia with high AC/A ratio (convergence excess). *J Pediatr Ophthalmol Strabismus.* 1985;22:238.

NONACCOMMODATIVE OR PARTIALLY ACCOMMODATIVE ESOTROPIA

Epidemiology and Etiology

- Refractive or nonrefractive accommodative esotropias do not always occur in their "pure" forms. Some patients may show no response to correction of their hyperopia. Other patients may have a significant reduction in esodeviation when given glasses, but a residual esodeviation persists despite full hyperopic correction. Still others may show an initial good response only to develop a crossing that can no longer be completely corrected with glasses. The crossing not corrected with the glasses is the nonaccommodative portion. This condition commonly occurs when there is a delay of months between the onset of accommodative esotropia and antiaccommodative treatment.

Signs and Symptoms

- Patients with nonaccommodative esotropia have little or no hyperopia. They may also have a level of hyperopia that does not appear compatible with the degree of crossing.
- Patients with a partial accommodative esotropia appear to have a level of hyperopia that

will correct their crossing. However, they do not demonstrate a resolution of their crossing when wearing their glasses.

Differential Diagnosis

- Congenital esotropia
- Accommodative esotropia

Diagnostic Evaluation

- A complete examination with cycloplegic refraction should be performed. If a significant level of hyperopia exists, the patient should be prescribed the full hyperopic correction and return after wearing glasses for a period of time.

Treatment

- If the nonaccommodative component of the crossing is large enough to prevent the development of binocular vision, strabismus surgery should be considered. Some surgeons will not opt for surgery if the crossing is small and not easily noticed.

Prognosis

- Patients with small levels of hyperopia may be able to discontinue wearing their glasses. Recurrent strabismus is possible in these patients, who often have abnormal binocular vision even after successful treatment.

CONGENITAL EXOTROPIA

Epidemiology and Etiology

- Congenital exotropia behaves in a very similar fashion to congenital esotropia. It typically occurs early in life and presents with a large, constant out-turning. Congenital exotropia may be associated with neurologic disease or abnormalities of the bony orbit, as in Crouzon's syndrome.

Signs and Symptoms

- Patients with congenital exotropia often appear to have decreased adduction on side gaze; with gaze right or left, the abducting eye fixates while the opposite eye approaches midline and stops. This is similar to the cross fixation found in children with congenital esotropia. Occlusion or the doll's head maneuver will demonstrate that good adduction is possible.

- Amblyopia is not common because these children typically alternate fixation. The refractive error is similar to that of the general population.

Differential Diagnosis

- Early-onset intermittent exotropia
- Third cranial nerve palsy
- Bilateral intranuclear ophthalmoplegia

Diagnostic Evaluation

- A complete examination should be performed.
- Other signs of a cranial nerve palsy (ptosis, decreased motility) should be eliminated.

Treatment

- Patients with congenital constant exotropia are operated on early in life in the same manner as patients with congenital esotropia.

Prognosis

- Similar to patients with congenital esotropia, early surgery in these patients can lead to gross binocular vision but not bifoveal fixation.
- These patients also tend to develop DVD and IOOA and should be followed closely for the development of these associated motility disturbances.

REFERENCE

Hunter DG, Kelly JB, Buffenn AN, et al. Long-term outcome of uncomplicated infantile exotropia. *J AAPOS*. 2001;5:352–356.

INTERMITTENT EXOTROPIA

Epidemiology and Etiology

- Intermittent exotropia is the most common exodeviation in childhood.
- The etiology of intermittent exotropia is unknown but probably results from a combination of mechanical and innervational factors.

Signs and Symptoms

- The age of onset of intermittent exotropia varies but is often between age 6 months and 4 years.
- It is characterized by outward drifting of one eye, which usually occurs when a child is fixating at distance (Fig. 9-7). The deviation is generally more frequent with fatigue or illness. Exposure to bright light may cause reflex closure of the exotropic eye.
- Because the deviation generally begins with distance fixation and is only seen when the child is tired, it is often not seen when the child is examined by a primary medical doctor at close distance or during a well-child visit.

Differential Diagnosis

- Congenital exotropia

Diagnostic Evaluation

- A complete evaluation should be performed. Motility measurements at both distance and near fixation should be completed. A qualitative measurement of the control of the strabismus should be noted.

Treatment

- Any coexistent amblyopia should be treated. Significant refractive errors should be corrected. Some ophthalmologists use medical treatments to avoid surgery in some patients. These nonsurgical treatments include part-time occlusion, orthoptic therapy, and over minus lens therapy. Most patients eventually require strabismus surgery when the deviation becomes manifest frequently.

Prognosis

- Surgery is successful in aligning most patients' eyes. Some patients will redevelop strabismus and may require more surgery.

REFERENCE

Kushner BJ. Exotropic deviations: a functional classification and approach to treatment. *Am Orthoptic J.* 1988;38:81–93.

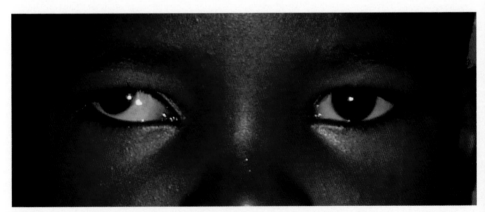

FIGURE 9-7. Intermittent exotropia demonstrating manifest exotropia at distance fixation.

A AND V PATTERN STRABISMUS

Epidemiology and Etiology

- A and V patterns are manifested by a horizontal change of alignment as the eyes move from the primary position to midline upgaze or downgaze.

- A number of different theories have evolved to explain the etiology of A and V patterns. There is no universal agreement of their cause at this time.

- Oblique muscle dysfunction is often seen in the setting of A and V pattern strabismus (Figs. 9-8 and 9-9). The oblique muscles have secondary abducting action. Therefore, when the superior obliques are overacting, they may cause an A pattern; when the inferior obliques are overacting or the superior obliques are underacting, a V pattern often results. However, A and V patterns frequently exist in the absence of demonstrable oblique dysfunction.

Signs and Symptoms

- Esotropia with V pattern increases in downgaze and decreases in upgaze. The deviation in V exotropia increases in upgaze and decreases in downgaze.

- In A esotropia, the deviation increases in upgaze and decreases in downgaze.

- In A exotropia, the deviation increases in downgaze and decreases in upgaze.

- Anomalous head posture is common in patients with A and V patterns.

- Patients with A esotropia and V exotropia and fusion in downgaze may develop a chin-up position. Conversely, V esotropia and A exotropia may cause chin depression.

Differential Diagnosis

- A and V pattern strabismus should be looked for in patients with compensatory chin-up or chin-down strabismus.

- Restrictive or paralytic strabismus may also present with abnormal head postures.

- Brown's syndrome may manifest a V pattern.

Diagnostic Evaluation

- The A and V patterns are demonstrated by measuring a deviation in primary position and in approximately 25 degrees of upgaze and downgaze while the patient fixates on a distant object.

- An A pattern is said to exist if divergence increases in downgaze by 10 or more prism diopters.

- A V pattern signifies an increase in divergence of 15 or more prism diopters in upgaze. The smaller amount of change required to make a diagnosis of an A pattern is caused by the greater effect of the downgaze deviation on reading and other near tasks.

Treatment

- Patients with torticollis may benefit from treatment. Patients with large patterns often have significant oblique dysfunction. Treatment of the oblique dysfunction is usually needed to treat these large patterns. However, superior oblique weakening should be done with extreme caution is patients with A pattern strabismus and good binocular function because an asymmetric result can lead to permanent torsional diplopia. In patients without oblique dysfunction, vertically moving or offsetting the horizontal rectus muscle weakens the action of that muscle when the eye is moved in the direction of the offsetting. For example, if the medial rectus muscles are moved up one-half tendon width, their horizontal action further decreases in upgaze. Therefore, moving the medial rectus toward the apex of an A and V pattern or moving the lateral rectus muscle toward the open end of the A or V is appropriate for correcting the incomitant deviation. This is true regardless of whether recession or resection is performed. The tendon is generally moved up or down half of its insertion width.

Prognosis

- Surgery is generally effective is collapsing the pattern and decreasing or eliminating the associated head posture when present.

REFERENCE

Scott WE, Drummond GT, Keech RV. Vertical offsets of horizontal recti muscles in the management of A and V pattern strabismus. *Aust N Z J Ophthalmol.* 1989;17:281.

Knapp P. Vertically incomitant horizontal strabismus: The so called A and V Syndrome. *Trans Am Ophthalmol Soc.* 1959;57:666–698.

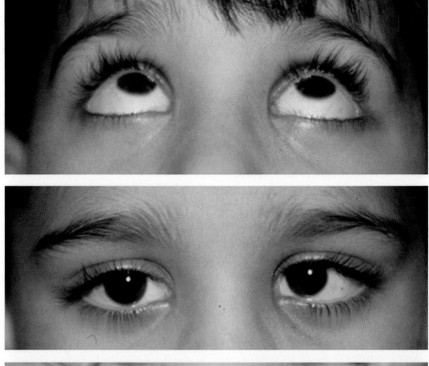
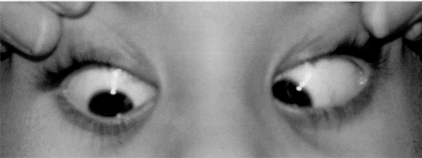

FIGURE 9-8. V pattern esotropia. The esotropia increase in straight down gaze and decreases in straight up gaze.

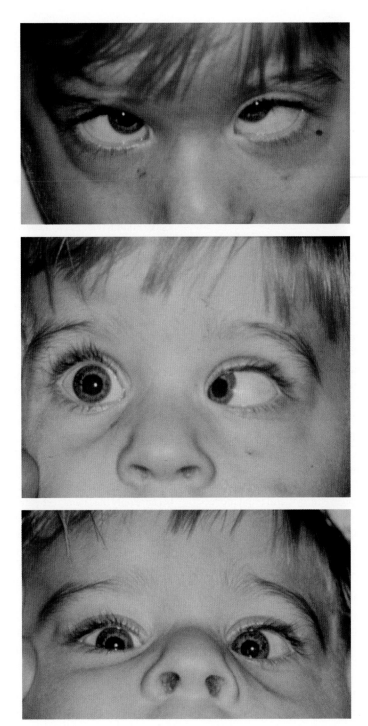

FIGURE 9-9. A pattern esotropia. The esotropia increases in straight up gaze and decreases in straight down gaze.

THIRD NERVE PALSY

Epidemiology and Etiology

• In children, third nerve palsies are usually congenital. The congenital form is often associated with a developmental anomaly or birth trauma. Acquired third nerve palsies can be an ominous sign and may indicate a neurologic abnormality such as an intracranial neoplasm or an aneurysm. Other less serious causes include an inflammatory or infectious lesion, head trauma, postviral syndromes, and migraines.

Signs and Symptoms

• A third nerve palsy, whether congenital or acquired, usually results in an exotropia and a hypotropia of the affected eye, as well as complete or partial ptosis of the upper eyelid (Fig. 9-10A). This characteristic strabismus results from the action of the normal, unopposed muscles, the lateral rectus muscle and the superior oblique muscle. If the internal branch of the third nerve is involved, pupillary dilation may be noted as well. Adduction, elevation, and depression are usually limited (Fig. 9-10B).

• In congenital and traumatic cases of third nerve palsy, a misdirection of regenerating nerve fibers may develop, referred to as *aberrant regeneration*. This results in anomalous and paradoxical eyelid, eye, and pupil movement such as elevation of the eyelid, constriction of the pupil, or depression of the globe on attempted adduction.

Differential Diagnosis

• Congenital exotropia

• Congenital fibrosis of the extraocular muscles (CFEOM)

Diagnostic Evaluation

• Diagnosis is based on the characteristic exotropia and hypotropia with associated limitation in adduction and vertical movements of the eye.

• Pupillary involvement is an especially important sign because it may indicate an expanding intracranial aneurysm and need for emergent neurologic evaluation and treatment.

• Patients with an acquired third nerve palsy should have a neurologic evaluation, including neuroimaging when indicated.

Treatment

• Initial treatment for patients with acquired third nerve palsy involves relief of diplopia. If there is complete third nerve palsy, the associated complete ptosis will cover the pupil and prevent diplopia. However, in partial third nerve palsy, the eyelid may not cover the pupillary space, so diplopia may remain a problem. Occlusion therapy is then the best solution for the diplopia. In children young enough to develop amblyopia, the patch should be alternated so the affected eye will continue to develop normal vision.

• Surgery to correct acquired third nerve palsy should be postponed for several months after the onset of the condition when possible. If the ptosis is complete and the eyelid cannot open, early ptosis surgery may be needed in younger children to prevent the development of amblyopia. In a complete third nerve palsy, the motility of the globe is severely limited because only the lateral rectus and superior oblique muscles are functional. Surgical options include lateral rectus recession, superior oblique weakening or transposition, and fixation of the globe to the orbital wall with a nonabsorbable suture or fascia lata.

Prognosis

• The goal of surgical intervention is to use the two remaining functional muscles in such a way as to achieve a straight-ahead eye with only limited movement of the globe. This goal should be carefully explained to the patient and parents to avoid unrealistic postoperative expectations.

REFERENCES

Holmes JM, Mutyala S, Maus TL, et al. Pediatric third, fourth, and sixth nerve palsies: a population-based study. *Am J Ophthalmol.* 1999;127:388–392.

Keane JR. Third nerve palsy: analysis of 1400 personally-examined inpatients. *Can J Neurol Sci.* 2010;37:662–670.

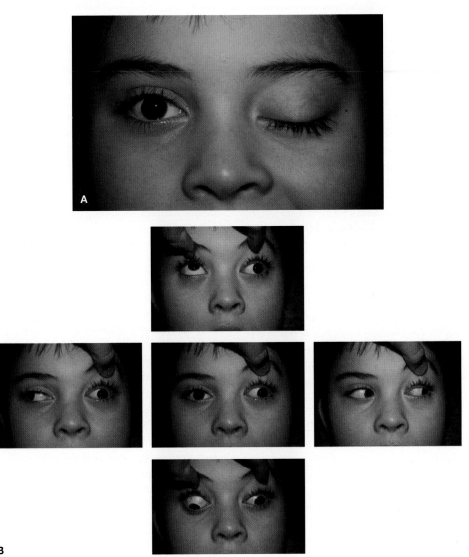

FIGURE 9-10. Third nerve palsy. (From Nelson LB, Olitsky SE. *A Color Handbook of Pediatric Clinical Ophthalmology.* London: Manson Publishing; 2011.)

FOURTH NERVE PALSY

Epidemiology and Etiology

- Fourth nerve palsy is the most common cause of an isolated cyclovertical muscle palsy. Paresis of the fourth nerve can be congenital or acquired. Closed-head trauma is the most common cause of acquired fourth nerve palsy and other causes include cerebrovascular accident, diabetes, brain tumor, ethmoiditis, or mastoiditis.

Signs and Symptoms

- Patients with unilateral fourth nerve palsy often present with torticollis to reduce diplopia. This usually consists of a head tilt to the side of the nonparetic eye, a face turn to the contralateral side, and a small chin-down head posture. Patients with a bilateral palsy usually place their heads in a chin-down position.

- The absence of a head tilt in a preverbal child should raise the suspicion of amblyopia.

- Facial asymmetry has been associated with congenital superior oblique palsy and typically is manifested by midfacial hemihypoplasia on the dependent side opposite the affected superior oblique. The nose deviates toward the hypoplastic side, and the mouth slants so that it approximates a horizontal orientation despite the torticollis.

Differential Diagnosis

- Any vertical strabismus that leads to a hypertropia

Diagnostic Evaluation

- To evaluate a suspected fourth nerve palsy, a three-step test should be performed. A patient with a fourth nerve palsy will demonstrate a hypertropia that is worse when looking to the contralateral side and when the head is tilted to the ipsilateral side of the affected eye (Fig. 9-11).

- When a patient presents with a new onset of diplopia secondary to a fourth nerve palsy, it is important to determine if the palsy has only recently developed or if it represents a congenital disorder that has decompensated. Several features may help to determine the acuteness of the deviation. A patient with a congenital superior oblique palsy will often have large vertical fusional amplitudes and a longstanding head tilt that can be documented in old photographs. Facial asymmetry may be present.

- In patients with a fourth nerve palsy, bilateral involvement should be excluded. Signs of bilateral fourth nerve palsy include hypertropia that alternates in right and left gaze and in right and left head tilt, a V pattern esotropia, and a large degree of excyclotorsion on either double Maddox rod testing or funduscopic evaluation.

Treatment

- Except for an occasional patient with a fairly comitant vertical deviation of 10 prism diopters or less (when prism may be tolerated), most cases of superior oblique palsy require surgery. In general, surgery for superior oblique palsies should be directed to those muscles whose greatest action is in the field when the vertical deviation is the largest. Surgical options include superior oblique tuck, inferior oblique weakening, ipsilateral superior rectus recession or contralateral inferior rectus recession, or various combinations of these procedures.

Prognosis

- Surgical treatment is helpful in reducing or eliminating the abnormal head posture, normalizing ocular rotations, and enlarging the area of single binocular vision in most patients.

REFERENCES

Morris RJ, Scott WE, Keech RV. Superior oblique tuck surgery in the management of superior oblique palsies. *J Pediatr Ophthalmol Strabismus.* 1992;29:337.

Parks MM. Isolated cyclovertical muscle palsy. *Arch Ophthalmol.* 1958;60:1027.

Wilson ME, Hoxie J. Facial asymmetry in superior oblique muscle palsy. *J Pediatr Ophthalmol Strabismus.* 1993;30:315.

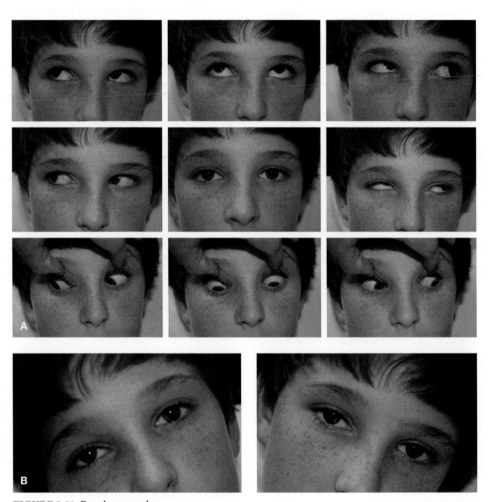

FIGURE 9-11. Fourth nerve palsy.

SIXTH NERVE PALSY

Epidemiology and Etiology

- Sixth nerve palsies can be congenital or acquired (Fig. 9-12). Congenital sixth nerve palsies are rare. Acquired sixth nerve palsy is more common.

- The sixth nerve has a long intracranial course, and there are three anatomic areas where the sixth nerve is most susceptible to injury: (1) as it exits from the pontomedullary junction (2) at its penetration of the dura (Dorello's canal) and (3) within the cavernous sinus.

- Trauma is probably the most common cause of an acquired sixth nerve palsy. Other causes include neoplastic, inflammatory, vascular, and postviral. Acquired bilateral sixth nerve palsy is usually a manifestation of a serious intracranial abnormality or an increase in intracranial pressure (ICP).

Signs and Symptoms

- Patients with an acute sixth nerve palsy usually present with diplopia. If the palsy is unilateral, double vision may be avoided by adopting a compensatory head posture with the eyes in the lateral gaze position away from the palsied eye; this results in a compensatory horizontal face turn toward the palsied eye.

Differential Diagnosis

- Congenital esotropia
- Duane's syndrome
- Mobius syndrome

Diagnostic Evaluation

- A complete examination should be performed, and signs of increased ICP (papilledema) should be sought. Neurologic consultation and neuroimaging should be considered for most patients. A lumbar puncture may be needed to document increased ICP.

- Most patients with suspected congenital sixth nerve palsy have congenital esotropia with cross-fixation of one or both eyes. It is important to identify these patients to avoid unnecessary diagnostic procedures.

Treatment

- Initial treatment may consist of occlusion to eliminate diplopia. Children with significant hyperopia should be given glasses to avoid the development of an accommodative esotropia. If the deviation does not improve over time, surgery may be necessary.

- If there is lateral rectus function, a unilateral medial rectus recession combined with a lateral rectus resection can be performed.

- If little or no function of the lateral rectus exists, a transposition procedure may be needed.

Prognosis

- Many patients can be given single vision in with or without a small face turn. Patients should understand that the range of single binocular vision may be limited; this is especially true in bilateral cases.

REFERENCES

Brooks SE, Olitsky SE, deB Ribeiro G. Augmented Hummelsheim procedure for paralytic strabismus. *J Pediatr Ophthalmol Strabismus.* 2000;37:189–195.

Holmes JM, Beck RW, Kip KE, et al. Botulinum toxin treatment versus conservative management in acute traumatic sixth nerve palsy or paresis. *J AAPOS.* 2000; 4:145–149.

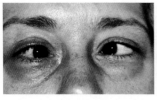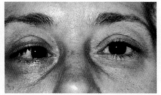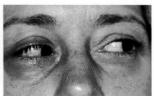

FIGURE 9-12. Sixth nerve palsy.

DUANE'S SYNDROME

Epidemiology and Etiology

- Duane's syndrome is found in approximately 1% of individuals with strabismus. It occurs more frequently in the left eye than in the right and in females more than in males.

- Bilateral involvement is less frequent than unilateral occurrence (Fig. 9-13).

- Although Duane's syndrome has been well described clinically, the etiology remains unclear. Various theories include structural and innervational anomalies of the extraocular muscles as well as absence or hypoplasia of the sixth nerve nucleus.

- Up- and downshoots that may be seen in Duane's syndrome may occur because of co-innervation of the horizontal and vertical rectus muscles or slippage of the lateral rectus muscle above or below the eye, commonly referred to as a "leash phenomenon."

Signs and Symptoms

- The most characteristic clinical findings in Duane's syndrome include an absence of abduction of an eye with slight limitation of adduction, retraction of the globe in attempted adduction, and up- and down-shooting or both in adduction. Classically, Duane's syndrome has been grouped into three types:

  - Type I: marked limitation or complete absence of abduction; normal or only slightly restricted adduction

  - Type II: limitation or absence of adduction with exotropia of the affected eye; normal or slightly limited abduction

  - Type III: severe limitation of both abduction and adduction

- Other ocular or systemic anomalies are commonly seen in patients with Duane's syndrome. Ocular anomalies may include dysplasia of the iris stroma, pupillary anomalies, cataracts, heterochromia, Marcus Gunn jaw winking, coloboma, crocodile tears, and microphthalmos. The systemic anomalies include Goldenhar syndrome; dystrophic defects such as the Klippel-Feil syndrome; cervical spina bifida; cleft palate; facial anomalies; perceptive deafness; malformations of the external ear; and anomalies of the limbs, feet, and hands.

Differential Diagnosis

- Sixth nerve palsy
- Congenital esotropia
- Exotropia

Diagnostic Evaluation

- The disorder most commonly confused with Duane's syndrome is sixth nerve palsy. Patients with a sixth nerve palsy generally have a much larger deviation in primary position than patients with Duane's syndrome given the magnitude of the abduction deficit. In addition, an exotropia can usually be found in gaze to the opposite side in patients with Duane's syndrome and does not occur in sixth nerve palsies.

Treatment

- Before surgery is contemplated, coexisting significant refractive errors, anisometropia, and amblyopia should be treated. Indications for surgery include a significant deviation in primary position, an anomalous head position, a large up- or downshoot, or retraction of the globe that is cosmetically intolerable.

- Surgery usually involves recession of the medial or lateral rectus for patients with esotropia of exotropia. Some surgeons prefer transposition surgery. The medial rectus of the involved is usually tight, and forced duction testing results are often positive because of the contracture of the muscle.

- Resection of the ipsilateral lateral rectus should almost never be performed because it will increase retraction of the globe in adduction. If an up- or downshoot of the eye occurs, surgical options include recessing a stiff, fibrotic lateral rectus muscle, performing a Y splitting of the muscle, or placement of a posterior fixation suture to reduce the leash effect when present.

- Patients who have a cosmetically noticeable retraction of the globe in attempted adduction may benefit from recession of both horizontal recti to reduce the co-contraction. This can be done in the absence of a deviation in primary gaze or adjusted to eliminate a deviation if present.

Prognosis

- Surgery can help to reduce or eliminate an associated torticollis. Few patients show improvement in abduction after surgery, and some patients undergoing medial rectus recession may have a decrease in adduction.

- In patients with significant co-contraction, large overcorrections can occur after medial rectus recession.

REFERENCES

Huber A. Electrophysiology of the retraction syndrome. *Br J Ophthalmol.* 1974;59:293.

Pressman SH, Scott WE. Surgical treatment of Duane's syndrome. *Ophthalmology.* 1986;93:29.

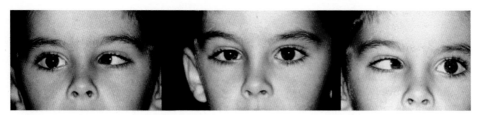

FIGURE 9-13. Bilateral Duane's syndrome.

BROWN'S SYNDROME

Epidemiology and Etiology

- Brown's syndrome may occur as a congenital or acquired defect and can be permanent, transient, or intermittent. Congenital Brown's syndrome occurs because of an anomaly of the anterior sheath of the superior oblique tendon. The acquired form has been attributed to a variety of causes, including superior oblique surgery, scleral buckling bands, trauma, and after sinus surgery and inflammation in the trochlear region.

- Brown's syndrome can be acquired in patients with juvenile or adult rheumatoid arthritis and represents a stenosing tenosynovitis of the trochlea that shares similar characteristics to inflammatory disorders that affect the tendons of the fingers.

Signs and Symptoms

- Brown's syndrome is characterized by a deficiency of elevation in the adducting position. Improved elevation is usually apparent in the midline, with normal or near-normal elevation in abduction (Fig. 9-14). With lateral gaze in the opposite direction, the involved eye may depress in adduction. Exodeviation (V pattern) often occurs as the eyes are moved upward in the midline. Many patients are orthophoric in primary position.

- If a hypotropia is present, the patient may develop a compensatory face turn toward the opposite eye.

- In some cases, there is discomfort on attempted elevation in adduction, the patient may feel or even hear a click under the same circumstances, and there may be a palpable mass or tenderness in the trochlear region.

A positive forced duction test result is the hallmark of Brown's syndrome.

Differential Diagnosis

- Inferior oblique palsy
- Superior oblique overaction
- Monocular elevation deficiency (MED)

Diagnostic Evaluation

- Patients will often display a V pattern, which helps distinguish Brown's syndrome from superior oblique overaction (A pattern).

- Forced duction testing should be performed; results are positive in individuals with Brown's syndrome.

Treatment

- Treatment is generally reserved for patients with a compensatory head posture, a hypotropia in primary position, or a large downshoot in adduction.

- Surgical treatment consists of a weakening procedure of the superior oblique tendon, which may include partial or full tenotomy, superior oblique recession, or superior oblique spacer.

- Patients with Brown's syndrome secondary to an inflammatory process may respond to corticosteroids or nonsteroidal anti-inflammatory agents given systemically as well as injection of corticosteroids into the trochlear region.

Prognosis

- Up to one-third of patients that undergo surgery superior oblique tenotomy develop an iatrogenic superior oblique palsy that may require further surgery.

- Even with successful surgery, elevation in adduction may continue to be abnormal in some patients.

REFERENCES

Helveston EM, Merriam WW, Ellis FD, et al. The trochlea. A study of the anatomy and physiology. *Ophthalmology.* 1982;89(2):124–133.

Parks MM, Eustis HS. Simultaneous superior oblique tenotomy and inferior oblique recession in Brown's syndrome. *Ophthalmology.* 1987;94:1043.

Wright KW. Superior oblique silicone expander for Brown's syndrome and superior oblique overaction. *J Pediatr Ophthalmol Strabismus.* 1991;28:101.

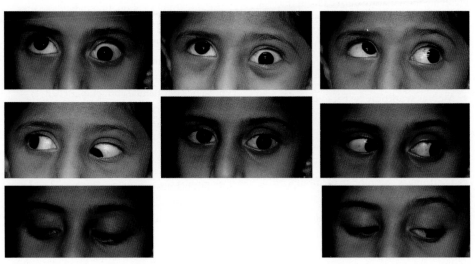

FIGURE 9-14. Acquired Brown's syndrome.

MÖBIUS SYNDROME

Epidemiology and Etiology

- Möbius syndrome is a rare congenital disturbance consisting of varying involvement of facial and lateral gaze paresis.

- The etiology of Möbius syndrome is presently unknown. Theories to explain this condition include a mesodermal dysplasia involving musculature derived from the first and second branchial arches or a vascular theory with disruption of blood flow during embryogenesis.

Signs and Symptoms

- Möbius syndrome is characterized by a unilateral or bilateral inability to abduct the eyes. Although horizontal movements are usually lacking, vertical movements and convergence are intact.

- Esotropia is common in children with Möbius syndrome (Fig. 9-15).

- Unilateral or bilateral complete or incomplete facial palsy is usually observed during the first few weeks of life because of difficulty with sucking and feeding and incomplete closure of the eyelids during sleep. These patients typically have masklike faces with an inability to grin and wrinkle the forehead.

Differential Diagnosis

- Congenital esotropia

- Bilateral cranial nerve six palsy

Diagnostic Evaluation

- Similar to that in congenital esotropia. Patients show an abduction deficit and may be forced duction positive on testing in the operating room.

- Most patients carry a diagnosis before seeing an ophthalmologist. However, the presence of bilateral abduction deficit, typical facial appearance, and difficulty feeding should prompt a further evaluation with a geneticist if a diagnosis has not been made.

Treatment

- Strabismus surgery is usually required to align the eyes. Transposition surgery is preferred by some ophthalmologists.

Prognosis

- Alignment in primary position is possible in most patients.

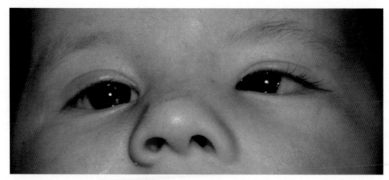

FIGURE 9-15. Möbius syndrome. (From Nelson LB, Olitsky SE. *A Color Handbook of Pediatric Clinical Ophthalmology*. London: Manson Publishing; 2011.)

MONOCULAR ELEVATION DEFICIENCY

Epidemiology and Etiology

- MED, formerly called double elevator palsy, suggests that both elevator muscles (the superior rectus and inferior oblique muscles) of one eye are weak, with a resultant inability or reduced ability to elevate the eye and a hypotropia in the primary position (Fig. 9-16). The term is generally used to describe diminished ocular elevation present in all fields of gaze.

- MED may be caused by innervational problems, restrictive conditions, or a combination of factors.

Signs and Symptoms

- Patients may present with a hypotropia or apparent ptosis. Some patients may develop a compensatory head posture with their chin in an upward position to maintain binocular vision.

- There is an inability elevate the eye in all fields of gaze.

- In patients in whom a restriction of upgaze is present, there may be an accentuated lower eyelid fold associated with inferior rectus restriction. This fold becomes more prominent with attempted upgaze.

Differential Diagnosis

- Brown's syndrome

- Thyroid-related strabismus with inferior rectus muscle restriction

- Orbital floor fracture with entrapment of the inferior rectus muscle

Diagnostic Evaluation

- The presence of a true ptosis should be ruled out by forcing the patient to fixate with the involved eye. In cases of pseudoptosis caused by the ipsilateral hypotropia, the ptosis will disappear when the eye is brought to midline.

- Forced duction testing is needed to eliminate a restricted inferior rectus muscle as the cause of the MED.

Treatment

- In cases of inferior rectus muscle restriction, the involved muscle should be recessed. When no restriction is present, a transposition procedure (Knapp procedure) is usually required.

Prognosis

- Alignment in primary position and reduction of the abnormal head posture are the goals of treatment.

- Elevation is not usually improved in cases involving a weakness of the elevator muscles.

REFERENCES

Metz HS. Double elevator palsy. *Arch Ophthalmol.* 1979;97:901.

Scott WE, Jackson OB. Double elevator palsy: the significance of inferior rectus restriction. *Am Orthop J* 1977;27:5.

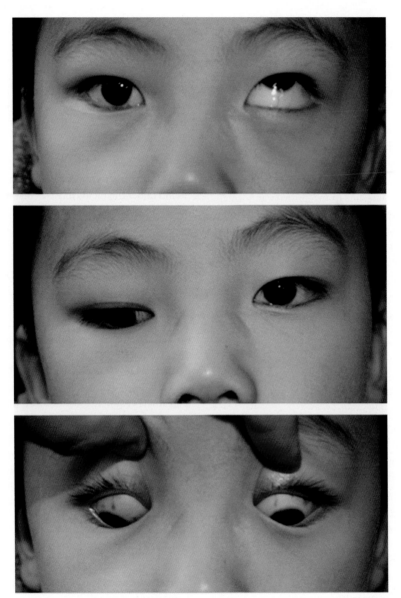

FIGURE 9-16. Monocular elevation deficiency of the right eye. Note the pseudoptosis of the right upper eyelid. (From Nelson LB, Olitsky SE. *A Color Handbook of Pediatric Clinical Ophthalmology*. London: Manson Publishing; 2011.)

CONGENITAL FIBROSIS OF THE EXTRAOCULAR MUSCLES

Epidemiology and Etiology

- CFEOM is a rare disease that occurs in approximately 1 in 230,000 people. Patients with CFEOM are usually born with ophthalmoplegia and ptosis (**Fig. 9-17**).

- Although the name of the syndrome suggests that it results from a primary abnormality of muscle, there is evidence that suggests that it may be result from a primary abnormality of the cranial nerve's innervation of these muscles.

- There are four subtypes of CFEOM, and the genes have been localized for three of them. Both autosomal dominant and autosomal recessive inheritance patterns have been observed.

Signs and Symptoms

- When evaluating an individual with suspected CFEOM, a thorough family history should be obtained.

- CFEOM is present at birth, is nonprogressive, and is frequently associated with ptosis. Depending on the subtype, it may be unilateral or bilateral.

- The specific position of the eyes and pattern of movement defines each clinical subtype of CFEOM.

Differential Diagnosis

- Double elevator palsy
- Third nerve palsy
- Chronic progressive ophthalmoplegia
- Thyroid-related strabismus

Diagnostic Evaluation

- A family history may reveal other relatives with a similar disorder. Genetic testing can confirm the diagnosis in some patients.

- Forced duction testing results are positive.

- During surgery, fibrotic bands can be found under the rectus muscles that must be located and severed to allow the eye to move during surgery.

Treatment

- The goal of surgical management in the general fibrosis syndrome is to center the eyes and improve the compensatory head posture. In patients with significant hypotropia, large recession or disinsertion of the inferior rectus muscles is indicated. However, elevation of the hypotropic eye accentuates the ptosis. Bilateral frontalis suspension is required soon after the strabismus surgery.

- Because these patients often do not have a Bell's phenomenon, corneal drying may occur after ptosis surgery. Therefore, the eyelid should be elevated only to the upper pupillary border.

Prognosis

- These are very challenging patients and may require multiple surgeries to help reduce their compensatory head posture to provide comfortable vision.

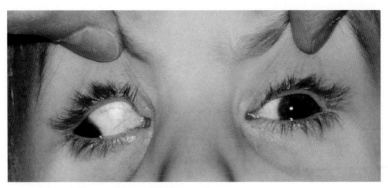

FIGURE 9-17. Congenital fibrosis of the extraocular muscles.

Index

NOTE: Page numbers followed by 'f' and 't' refer figures and tables respectively.

A

A and V pattern strabismus, 185–186, 187f
AAV. *see* Adeno-associated viral (AAV)
Abetalipoproteinemia, 146
Abnormalities affecting eye
  anophthalmia, 2–7
  microphthalmia, 8–11
  nanophthalmia, 12–13
Accommodative esotropia, 182
Achromatopsia, 116
Acquired corneal cloudiness, 24
Acquired corneal pannus, 74
Acquired pupillary margin cysts, 72
Acyclovir, 38
Adeno-associated viral (AAV), 116
Adult foveomacular dystrophy, 111
Advanced retinitis pigmentosa, 112
Aicardi, 8
Alagille syndrome, 70
Alport's syndrome, 98
Amblyopia, 102, 108, 176
Angle-closure glaucoma, 59
Aniridia, 68–69f, 74–75f, 98, 102
Anisocoria, 65
Ankyloblepharon, 152–153f
Anophthalmia, 2–7
  clinical, 7f
  diagnosis, 3
  etiology, 2
  external examination of, 5f
  MRI of, 6f
  prognosis, 4
  signs and symptoms, 2–3
  treatment, 3–4
Anophthalmos, 2
Anterior lenticonus, 104–105f
Anterior or posterior lens dislocation, 108
Anterior polar cataract, 100f
Anterior segment dysgenesis, 55, 98
Anterior staphyloma, 32–33f
Antiglaucoma medications, 49
Antihistamine, 46
Anti- VEGF drug bevacizumab, 144
A pattern esotropia, 187f
Apert's disease, 102

Aphakic glaucoma, 55–56, 57f
Astigmatism, 20
Astigmatism, irregular, 108
Astrocytic hamartoma, 118–119, 119f
Axenfeld-rieger anomaly, 96–97f
Axenfeld-Rieger spectrum, 59, 65, 68, 70
  syndrome, 78

B

BAL. *see* British anti-Lewisite (BAL)
Bassen-Kornzweig syndrome, 116
Batten's disease, 150
Bestrophinopathy, 150
Best's disease, 110–111, 111f
Bilateral congenital mydriasis, 68
Bilateral cranial nerve six palsy, 198
Bilateral intranuclear ophthalmoplegia, 183
Biliary cirrhosis, 34
Birth trauma, 20
  Descemet's membrane ruptures, 21f
Birth trauma, forceps, 49
Blepharophimosis syndrome, 154–155f
  child with, 155f
Blurred vision, 168
Bone marrow transplant, 24
Bourneville's disease, 118
BPES, 166
Branch retinal artery occlusion, 148
British anti-Lewisite (BAL), 34
Brown's syndrome, 185, 196–197f, 200
  acquired, 197f
Brushfield spots, 76–77f, 86, 88
Bulging opacified cornea, 32
Buphthalmos and corneal clouding, 51f

C

Capillary hemangiomas, 62, 168–169f
Cataract, 74, 143
  extraction, 147
Central corneal leukoma, 26
Central corneal opacity, 26

Central pupillary cysts, 72–73f
CFEOM. *see* Congenital fibrosis of extraocular muscles (CFEOM)
CHARGE syndrome, 8, 14, 82
CHED. *see* Congenital hereditary endothelial dystrophy (CHED)
Chickenpox, 44–45f
Choriocapillaris, 114
Chorioretina, 14
  scars, 134
Chorioretinitis, 112, 114
Choroidal atrophy, 114
Choroidal hemangioma, 63–64f
Choroidal melanoma, 134
Choroideremia, 112–113, 113f, 114
Chronic active hepatitis, 34
Chronic iridocyclitis, 80
Chronic progressive ophthalmoplegia, 202
CHRPE, 134–135f
CHSD. *see* Congenital hereditary stromal dystrophy (CHSD)
Ciliary body
  cysts, 72
  tumors, 84
Coats' disease, 125–127f, 138, 143
  with mild temporal macular exudation, 126f
  skin findings in, 123f
  with xanthochroia, 127f
Coloboma, 162–163f
  abnormalities affecting eye, 14–17
  ankyloblepharon, 153f
  atypical, 14
  congenital, 152
  diagnosis, 14
  etiology, 14
  eyelid anomalies, 162–163f
  iris, 16f–17f, 82–83f
  iris anomalies, 82–83f
  prognosis, 15
  signs, 14
  treatment, 14
  unilateral and bilateral iris, 83f
  upper eyelid, 163f

Cone dystrophy, 116, 150
Congenital and acquired
    hypopigmented irides, 80
Congenital and developmental
    cataracts, 98–99, 100f–101f
Congenital corneal opacity
    anterior staphyloma, 32–33f
    birth trauma, 20–21f
    chickenpox, 44–45f
    corneal dermoid, 30–31f
    hepatolenticular degeneration,
        34–35f
    hereditary endothelial dystrophy,
        28–29f
    herpes simplex infection, 36–37f
    herpes simplex virus epithelial
        dendrite, 38–39f
    herpes zoster ophthalmicus, 42–43f
    HSV corneal stromal disease,
        40–41f
    limbal vernal keratoconjunctivitis,
        46–47
    mucopolysaccharidosis, 24–25f
    Peters' anomaly, 26–27f
    sclerocornea, 18–19f
    ulcer, 22–23f
Congenital ectropion, 65, 156–157f,
    162
    uveae, 65–66, 67f
Congenital entropion, 156, 158–159f
Congenital esotropia, 176–177f, 180,
    182, 192, 194, 198
Congenital exotropia, 183–184, 188
Congenital fibrosis, 203f
Congenital fibrosis of extraocular
    muscles (CFEOM), 188,
    202–203f
Congenital glaucoma, 102
Congenital hereditary endothelial
    dystrophy (CHED), 18, 20,
    28–29f, 49
Congenital hereditary stromal
    dystrophy (CHSD), 49
Congenital hypertrophy of retinal
    pigment epithelium, 135f
Congenital mucocele, 170–171f
Congenital nuclear cataract, 100f
Congenital nystagmus, 74
Congenital ptosis, 154, 160–161f
Congenital pupillary margin
    epithelial cysts, 72
Congenital sixth nerve palsy, 176
Congenital synechia, 94
Congenital syphilis, 102

Congenital tarsal kink, 156
Conjunctival nevi, 90
Contralateral microphthalmia, 49
Copper-deficient diet, 34
Corectopia, 78, 82
Corneal dermoid, 30–31f
Corneal edema, bilateral
    symmetrical, 28
Corneal haze, 28
Corneal hysteresis, 49
Corneal opacification, 21f
Corneal opacity, 40f
Cornea plana, 70
Corneoscleral transplant, 32
Cosmetic deformities, 4
Cotton wool patches, 148
Cryptophthalmos, 3, 152
Cutis marmorata telangiectasia
    congenita, 63
CYP1B1 (2p21) gene, 48
Cystic eye, 3
Cystinosis, 146
Cystoid macular edema, 140
Cytomegalovirus, 98

D

Dermis fat grafting, 4
Dermoid, 18, 20, 170
Descemet's membrane, 19f
Descemet's tears, 20
Diabetes mellitus, 98
Diffuse choroidal hemangioma, 62
Dilated tortuous conjunctival and
    episcleral vessels, 64f
Disciform keratitis, 40–41f, 42
Dissociated vertical deviation
    (DVD), 177f, 178–179,
    179f
Double elevator palsy, 200, 202
D-penicillamine, 34
Duane's retraction syndrome, 176
Duane's syndrome, 178, 192,
    194–195f
    bilateral, 195f
DVD. *see* Dissociated vertical
    deviation (DVD)
Dysmorphic syndromes, 146
Dystrophy
    adult foveomacular, 111
    cone, 116, 150
    hereditary endothelial, 28–29f
    juvenile retinal, 116
    myotonic, 98
    pattern, 110

E

Early-onset intermittent exotropia,
    183
Ecotopia lentis et pupillae, 78–79f
Ectopia
    lentis, 74, 102–103f
    lentis et pupillae, 92
    pupil, 82, 96
Ectropion, 157f
    syndrome, 80
Ehlers-Danlos syndrome, 102
Encephalocele, 170
Entropion, 164
Enzyme replacement, 24
Epiblepharon, 152, 158, 164–165f
Epicanthus, 154, 158, 166–167f
    tarsalis, 167f
ERFP. *see* Extraretinal fibrovascular
    proliferation (ERFP)
Esotropia
    accommodative, 182
    congenital, 176–177f, 182, 192,
        194, 198
    nonaccommodative, 180
    nonrefractive accommodative,
        180–181
    partially accommodative, 182
    A pattern, 187f
    refractive accommodative, 180–
        180f, 181
    sensory, 176–177f
    V pattern, 187f
Euryblepharon, 156, 162
Extraretinal fibrovascular
    proliferation (ERFP), 142
Eyelid anomalies
    ankyloblepharon, 152–153f
    blepharophimosis syndrome,
        154–155f
    capillary hemangiomas, 168–169f
    colobomas, 162–163f
    congenital ectropion, 156–157f
    congenital entropion, 158–159f
    congenital ptosis, 160–161f
    epiblepharon, 164–165f
    epicanthus, 166–167f

F

Fabry's disease, 98
Facial hemihypertrophy, 65
Facio auricular vertebral syndrome,
    30
Familial adenomatous polyposis
    (FAP), 134

Familial exudative vitreoretinopathy (FEVR), 120, 136–137f
Fanconi's syndrome, 146
FAP. *see* Familial adenomatous polyposis (FAP)
FEVR. *see* Familial exudative vitreoretinopathy (FEVR)
Fibrinous anterior uveitis, 92
Forceps injury, 70
Fourth nerve palsy, 190–191f
Frizzled 4 gene *(FZD4)*, 124
Fundus albipunctata, 150
Fundus flavimaculata, 150–151f

G

Galactosemia, 98
Ganciclovir ophthalmic gel, 38
Genetic counseling, 147, 151
Ghost cell glaucoma, 59
Gillespie syndrome, 68
Glaucoma, 18, 20, 74
   aniridia, 68–69f
   aphakic glaucoma, 55–56, 57f
   associated with anterior segment dysgenesis, 52
   congenital ectropion uveae, 65–66, 67f
   drainage devices, 59
   JOAG, 52–53, 54f
   posterior embryotoxon, 70–71f
   primary congenital, 48–50, 51f
   secondary to uveitis, 52
   Sturge-Weber syndrome, 62–63, 64f
   traumatic, 55, 59
   uveitic glaucoma, 58–60, 61f
Goldenhar syndrome, 2, 8
Goldman-Favre disease, 116, 140
Goltz, 8
Gyrate atrophy, 112, 114–115, 115f

H

Haab striae, 49, 51f, 70
Hallerman-Streiff, 2
Hemangioma, 170
Hepatolenticular degeneration, 34–35f
Herpes simplex blepharitis, 37f
Herpes simplex corneal dendrite, 39f
Herpes simplex infection, 36–37f
Herpes simplex virus, 98
   epithelial dendrite, 38–39f
Herpes zoster ophthalmicus, 36, 42–43f

Heterochromia iridis, 14, 62, 80–81f
Homocystinuria, 102
Horner's syndrome, 160
HSV corneal stromal disease, 40–41f
Hurler's syndrome, 24–25f
Hyperlysinemia, 102
Hyperopia, 9, 12
Hyperpigmented irides, 80
Hypertropia, 179
Hypopigmented elevated spots, 77f

I

Iatrogenic iris defect, 68
ICROP. *see* International classification of ROP (ICROP)
Incontinentia pigmenti, 121–122, 121t, 123f–124f, 136, 138, 143
Infantile glaucoma. *see also* Primary congenital
   child with, 50f
Infantile retinal nonattachment, 120
Inferior oblique overaction, 178f, 179
Inferior oblique palsy, 196
Inflatable tissue expanders, 3
Injectable calcium hydroxylapatite, 4
Intermittent exotropia, 184
Intermittent strabismus, 174
International classification of ROP (ICROP), 142
Interstitial keratitis, 40–41f
Intrahepatic cholestasis of childhood, 34
Intraocular pressure (IOP), 30
IOP. *see* Intraocular pressure (IOP)
Iridocorneal endothelial syndrome, 65
Iridodonesis, 102
Iris
   anomalies
      aniridia, 74–75f
      axenfeld-rieger anomaly, 96–97f
      brushfield spots, 76–77f
      central pupillary cysts, 72–73f
      coloboma, 82–83f
      ecotopia lentis et pupillae, 78–79f
      heterochromia iridis, 80–81f
      juvenile xanthogranuloma, 86–87f
      lisch nodules, 88–89f
      ocular melanocytosis, 90–91f

      persistent pupillary membrane, 92–93f
      posterior synechiae, 94–95f
      stromal cysts, 84–85f
   coloboma, 16f–17f, 68, 78, 102
   mamillations, 76, 86, 88
   melanoma, 72
   nevi, 76, 88
   pigment epithelium, 67f
   stromal cysts, 72
   traumatic injury, 82

J

Jeune's syndrome, 146
JIA. *see* Juvenile idiopathic arthritis (JIA)
JOAG. *see* Juvenile open-angle glaucoma (JOAG)
Juvenile idiopathic arthritis (JIA), 58, 61f, 98
Juvenile open-angle glaucoma (JOAG), 52–53, 54f
Juvenile retinal dystrophy, 116
Juvenile retinoschisis, 140–141f
Juvenile xanthogranuloma (JXG), 76, 86–87f, 88
Juvenile X-linked retinoschisis, 141f
JXG. *see* Juvenile xanthogranuloma (JXG)

K

Kayser-Fleischer ring, 34–35f
Keratitis, 49
Keratopercipitates, 40
Klippel-Trenaunay-Weber syndrome, 62

L

Lacrimal anomalies
   congenital mucocele, 170–171f
   NLDO, 172–173f
Leber congenital amaurosis, 116–117f
Lens anomalies
   anterior lenticonus, 104–105f
   congenital and developmental cataracts, 98–99, 100f–101f
   ectopia lentis, 102–103f
   posterior lenticonus, 106–107f
   spherophakia, 108–109f
Lenticular myopia, 108
Leukemic infiltrates, 86
Leukocoria, 14, 131f, 148
   from retinoblastoma, 129

Limbal vernal, 47f
  keratoconjunctivitis, 46–47
Lisch nodules, 86, 88–89f
Liver transplantation, 34
Lymphangioma, 168

M

Malattia leventinese, 150
Malignancies, 98
Marcus-Gunn jaw wink, 160
Marfan's syndrome, 102
Mast cell stabilizers, 46
MED. *see* Monocular elevation
  deficiency (MED)
Megalocornea, 49
Melanosis oculi, 81f. *see also* Ocular
  melanocytosis
Mesodermal dysgenesis, 70, 96
Microcornea, 9
Microphthalmia, 8
  CHARGE, 8, 14, 82
  complex, 8
  with cyst, 11f
  diagnosis, 9
  etiology, 8
  MRI showing, 11f
  prognosis, 9
  pure, 8
  severe, 8
  signs and symptoms, 8–9
  single-gene disorders, 8
  treatment, 9
  unilateral, 10f
Microphthalmos, 3
Microspherophakia, 109f
Möbius syndrome, 176, 192,
  198–199f
Monocular elevation deficiency
  (MED), 196, 200–201f
Morning glory syndrome, 14
MPS. *see* Mucopolysaccharidosis
  (MPS)
Mucocele of nasolacrimal system,
  171f
Mucopolysaccharidosis (MPS), 20,
  24–25f, 49, 146
Myasthenia gravis, 160
Mydriatic drops, 59
Myelinated nerve fibers, 118, 148–149f
Myotonic dystrophy, 98

N

Nanophthalmia, 12
  bilateral, 13f

Nasal glioma, 170
Nasolacrimal duct obstruction
  (NLDO), 49, 172–173f
NDP gene. *see* Norrie's disease
  protein (NDP) gene
Neuroblastoma, 80
Neurofibromatosis, 65
Neuronal ceroid lipofuscinosis, 146
Nicotinic acid maculopathy, 140
NLDO. *see* Nasolacrimal duct
  obstruction (NLDO)
Nonaccommodative esotropia, 180
Nonrefractive accommodative
  esotropia, 180–181
Norrie's disease, 8, 138, 140
Norrie's disease protein (NDP) gene,
  124
Nyctalopia, 114
Nystagmus, 74, 82, 99

O

Ocular disorders, systemic and
  genetic basis of, 138t
Ocular melanocytosis, 80, 90–91f
Ocular prosthesis, 3, 9
Oculodermal melanocytosis, 80, 91f
Optic nerve
  granuloma, 118
  hypoplasia, 14
  pits, 14
Oral antihistamines, 46
Oral antiviral prophylaxis, 36
Orbital conformers, 9
Orbital dermoid, 168
Orbito-cranial advancement, 4
Ornithine aminotransferase gene
  (10q26), 114
Ovarian dysfunction, 154

P

Paralytic strabismus, 185
Partially accommodative esotropia,
  182
Pathologic myopia, 112
Pattern dystrophy, 110
PAX6 gene, 74
Peripheral anterior synechiae, 58, 70
Persistent fetal vasculature (PFV),
  124, 138–139f
Persistent hyperplastic primary
  vitreous (PHPV), 98, 124
Persistent pupillary membrane, 92–93f
Peters' anomaly, 18, 20, 26–27f, 49,
  70, 96

PFV. *see* Persistent fetal vasculature
  (PFV)
Phakomatosis pigmentovascularis, 63
Pharmacologic mydriasis, 68
Phenothiazines and chloroquine, 146
Photophobia, 74, 99
PHPV. *see* Persistent hyperplastic
  primary vitreous (PHPV)
Physiologic cupping, 52, 54f
Pigmented cysts, 73f
Pigment epithelial detachment, 111
Plasma ornithine levels, 114
Port wine mark, 63f
Posterior embryotoxon, 70–71f, 96
Posterior lenticonus, 106–107f
Posterior synechiae, 74, 94–95f
Prader-Willi syndrome, 65
Primary congenital, 48–50, 51f
Primary infantile glaucoma, 55, 62
Pseudoesotropia, 174–175f, 176
Pupillary block glaucoma, 102, 108
Pupillary margin epithelial cysts. *see*
  Central pupillary cysts

R

Rab escort protein 1 (REP-1), 112
Reactive hyperplasia, 134
Recurrent horizontal strabismus, 177
Refractive accommodative esotropia,
  180–180f, 181
Refsum's disease, 116, 146
Retinal anomalies
  astrocytic hamartoma, 118–119,
    119f
  best's disease, 110–111, 111f
  choroideremia, 112–113f
  CHRPE, 134–135f
  Coats' disease, 125–127f
  detachment from retinoblastoma,
    129
  dysplasia, 138
  familial exudative
    vitreoretinopathy, 136–137f
  fundus flavimaculata, 150–151f
  Gyrate atrophy, 114–115f
  incontinentia pigmenti, 121–122,
    123f–124f
  juvenile retinoschisis, 140–141f
  leber congenital amaurosis,
    116–117f
  myelinated nerve fibers, 148–149f
  persistent fetal vasculature,
    138–139f
  retinitis pigmentosa, 146–147f

retinoblastoma, 128–130, 131f–133f

retinopathy of prematurity, 142–144, 145f

Retinal pigment epithelium (RPE), 110

transplant, 147

Retinal toxoplasmosis, 14

Retinal vascular occlusion, 146

Retinitis pigmentosa, 102, 114, 146–147f

Retinitis punctate albescens, 150

Retinoblastoma, 128, 130–133f, 143

enucleation, 129

intraarterial chemotherapy, 129

intravenous chemoreduction, 129

Retinocytoma, 118

Retinopathy, solar, 110

Retinopathy of prematurity, 142–144, 144t, 145f

international classification of, 142t

Rhabdomyosarcoma, 168

Rhegmatogenous retinal detachment, 140

Rieger's syndrome, 102

RPE. *see* Retinal pigment epithelium (RPE)

Rubella, 98, 146

Rubeosis, 65

S

Scheie's syndrome, 24

Sclera, discoloration, 90

Sclerocornea, 18–19f, 20

Senior-Loken syndrome, 146

Sensory esotropia, 176–177f

Severe hypoplasia of iris, 75f

Sickle cell retinopathy, 136

Simple ectopia lentis, 102

Sixth nerve palsy, 192–193f, 194

Small-angle strabismus, 174

Sorsby's macular dystrophy, 110

Spherophakia, 102, 108–109f

Sporadic aniridia, 74

Staphyloma

enucleation specimen of, 33f

unilateral and bilateral anterior, 33f

Stargardt's disease, 110, 151f

Stellate congenital cataract, 101f

Steroid-induced glaucoma, 52, 59

Strabismus disorders, 74

Brown's syndrome, 196–197f

congenital esotropia, 176–177f

congenital exotropia, 183

congenital fibrosis of extraocular muscles, 202–203f

dissociated vertical deviation, 179

Duane's syndrome, 194–195f

fourth nerve palsy, 190–191f

inferior oblique overaction, 178f

intermittent exotropia, 184

Möbius syndrome, 198–199f

monocular elevation deficiency, 200–201f

nonrefractive accommodative esotropia, 181

partially accommodative esotropia, 182

pseudoesotropia, 174–175f

refractive accommodative esotropia, 180

sixth nerve palsy, 192–193f

third nerve palsy, 188–189f

A and V pattern strabismus, 185–186, 187f

Stromal cysts, 84–85f

Sturge-Weber syndrome, 62–63, 64f

Sulfite oxidase deficiency, 102

Superior oblique overaction, 196

Syphilis, 98

Systemic lupus erythematosus, 98

T

Tarsal kinking, 162

"Teardrop" pupil, 14

Tears in Descemet's membrane, 18

Third cranial nerve palsy, 183

Third nerve palsy, 160, 188–189f, 202

Thyroid-related strabismus, 200, 202

Topical antiglaucoma medications, 63

Toxocariasis, 138, 143

Toxoplasmosis, 98, 116

retinal, 14

Transient nevus flammeus of infancy, 62

Trauma, 65

to iris sphincter, 78

Trifluridine drops, 36, 38

True anophthalmia. *see* Anophthalmia

Tuberous Sclerosis, 118

U

Ulcer, 18, 20, 22

corneal, 23f

Unilateral and bilateral iris coloboma, 83f

Unilateral vesicular lesions, 42

Uveitic glaucoma, 55, 58–60, 61f

Uveitis, 42, 65

V

Valacyclovir, 38

Varicella, 98

Vesicular lesions on eyelid, 36

Vesicular rash, 42

Vitelliform macular dystrophy, 110

V pattern esotropia, 187f

W

Waardenburg syndromes, 2

Wagner's vitreoretinal dystrophy, 140

WAGR complex, 74

Walker- Warburg and Meckel-Gruber syndrome, 8

Weil-Marchesani syndrome, 102

Wilson's disease. *see* Hepatolenticular degeneration

Wolfflin nodules, 76

Y

YAG puncture. *see* Yttrium aluminium garnet (YAG) puncture

Yttrium aluminium garnet (YAG) puncture, 73

Z

Zellweger's syndrome, 146